Mental Healthcare in Brazilian Sp.
The Aesthetics of Healing

This volume addresses the diversification of mental healthcare provision and patients' health-seeking behavior by putting Brazilian Spiritism and its translocal relations at the center of its inquiry.

Comparative chapters document and critically assess the affective arrangements of Spiritist spaces in Brazil and Germany and how practices contribute to healing and the diversification of a globally circulating mental health agenda. This book addresses the human experience within Spiritist psychiatric clinics and affiliated Spiritist centers in Brazil, which in migratory contexts also have connections to Germany. Chapters interrogate the spaces where people inside and outside Brazil engage in implementing Spiritist practices in mental healthcare, introducing the Aesthetics of Healing as a conceptual tool to understand interactions between religion and medicine more broadly.

Establishing a novel analytical and interdisciplinary perspective on embodied aspects of sensory experience and perception, this compelling volume will be of interest to scholars, researchers, and postgraduate students involved with mental health research, medical anthropology, Spiritualism, and cross-cultural psychology. Practitioners in the fields of transcultural psychiatry and the sociology of religion will also find the volume of use.

Helmar Kurz is a Lecturer and Researcher in Medical Anthropology and Transcultural Psychiatry, currently associated with the Department of Social and Cultural Anthropology, University of Münster, Germany.

Explorations in Mental Health

Self and Identity
An Exploration of the Development, Constitution and Breakdown of Human Selfhood
Matthew Tieu

Co-Production in Mental Health
Implementing Policy into Practice
Michael Norton

Towards a Transtheoretical Definition of Countertransference
Re-visioning the Clinician's Intersubjective Experience
Rudy Roman

Challenging the Therapeutic Narrative
Historical and Clinical Perspectives on the Genetics of Behavior
Robert G. Goldstein

Critical Resilience and Thriving in Response to Systemic Oppression
Insights to Inform Social Justice in Critical Times
Melissa L. Morgan

Understanding Contemporary Diet Culture through the Lens of Lacanian Psychoanalytic Theor
Eating the Lack
Bethany Morris

Learning the Hard Way in Clinical Internships in Social Work and Psychology
Lessons for Safety, Boundary-Setting, and Deepening the Practicum Experience
Susan Lord

Mental Healthcare in Brazilian Spiritism: The Aesthetics of Healing
Helmar Kurz

For more information about this series, please visit www.routledge.com/Explorations-in-Mental-Health/book-series/EXMH

Mental Healthcare in Brazilian Spiritism: The Aesthetics of Healing

Helmar Kurz

Routledge
Taylor & Francis Group

LONDON AND NEW YORK

First published 2024
by Routledge
4 Park Square, Milton Park, Abingdon, Oxon OX14 4RN

and by Routledge
605 Third Avenue, New York, NY 10158

Routledge is an imprint of the Taylor & Francis Group, an informa business

British Library Cataloguing-in-Publication Data
A catalogue record for this book is available from the British Library

Library of Congress Cataloguing-in-Publication Data
Names: Kurz, Helmar, 1975- author.
Title: Mental healthcare in Brazilian spiritism : the aesthetics of healing / Helmar Kurz.
Description: Abingdon, Oxon ; New York, NY : Routledge, 2024. |
Series: Explorations in mental health | Includes bibliographical references and index. |
Identifiers: LCCN 2024001647 (print) | LCCN 2024001648 (ebook) | ISBN 9781032634173 (hardback) | ISBN 9781032637150 (paperback) | ISBN 9781032637167 (ebook)
Subjects: LCSH: Mental health services--Brazil. | Mental health--Religious aspects. | Spiritualism--Brazil. | Mental healing--Brazil. | Psychiatry and religion.
Classification: LCC RA790.7.B6 K87 2024 (print) | LCC RA790.7.B6 (ebook) | DDC 616.8/046520981--dc23/eng/20240222
LC record available at https://lccn.loc.gov/2024001647
LC ebook record available at https://lccn.loc.gov/2024001648

ISBN: 978-1-032-63417-3 (hbk)
ISBN: 978-1-032-63715-0 (pbk)
ISBN: 978-1-032-63716-7 (ebk)

DOI: 10.4324/9781032637167

Typeset in Sabon
by MPS Limited, Dehradun

TO MY UNCLE

Contents

Acknowledgments   *viii*
List of Abbreviations   *x*
List of Brazilian and Spiritist Expressions   *xi*
List of Figures   *xiv*

1   Introduction: Diversification of Mental Healthcare   1

2   Spiritism and Mental Health   25

3   Healing Cooperation: Therapeutic Spaces of Brazilian
    Spiritism   56

4   Aesthetics of Healing: A Sense of Self and Other   91

5   Translocal Networks and Politics of Care   122

6   Conclusion: Voices of Good Sense   154

References   *162*
Index   *180*

Acknowledgments

This book is a revised version of my PhD thesis in the disciplines of Ethnology and the Study of Religion, originally titled "Voices of Good Sense: Diversification of Mental Health and the Aesthetics of Healing in Brazilian Spiritism," designed as an Inaugural Dissertation, delivered on 17 November 2021, and successfully defended on 19 April 2022 at the Institute of Social and Cultural Anthropology, Department of History and Philosophy, University of Muenster/Germany. It analyzes data acquired within the research project Diversification of Mental Health: Therapeutic Spaces of Brazilian Spiritism initiated by Prof. Dr. Helene Basu and funded by the German Research Foundation DFG (Project Nr. 273588344). I, therefore, want to first thank DFG and Prof. Dr. Helene Basu for their support and accompaniment.

I want to further thank Prof. Dr. Andreas Hofbauer (*Departamento de Sociologia e Antropologia*, UNESP Marília, São Paulo, Brazil) for his mentorship throughout my research, and Prof. Dr. Bettina E. Schmidt (Institute for Education and Humanities, University of Wales, Trinity Saint David, UK) for enlightening discussions and her co-supervision. I also want to thank the Routledge team of the Mental Health Series for their professional support in bringing this book project to existence.

I want to thank all my interlocutors, colleagues, students, and "encounters," as well as my family and friends, for sharing, caring, listening, supporting, and trusting in me. I would need many extra pages to name all of them, but you all know that I am addressing YOU – both incarnate and disincarnate. In particular, I want to thank Michelle Drewke for reviewing my first manuscript and providing lovely support in finding the right words.

Last but surely not least, my eternal gratitude, bliss, and love are reserved for my, in every sense of the word, gorgeous companion, lover, and wife, Juliene. You made me do it!

Several aspects of this publication have already been discussed elsewhere (Kurz 2013, 2015, 2017, 2018a/b, 2019, 2022, 2023) but have been further elaborated and synthesized here to deliver a somewhat complete work that integrates my various experiences with Spiritist mental healthcare in Brazil and beyond and the divergent perspectives I have developed throughout over one decade of studying Spiritism and over 20 years of engaging with Brazilian culture.

Abbreviations

ABRAPE	Brazilian Association of Spiritist Psychologists
AME	Association of Spiritist Medicals
ASC	Altered States of Consciousness
ASSP	Altered States of Sensory Perception
CAM	Complementary and Alternative Medicines
CAPS	Psycho-Social Attention Center(s)
CEB	Spiritist Center Barsanulfo (Marília, SP, Brazil)
CECC	Spiritist Center House of the Path (Araraquara, SP, Brazil)
CECC	Spiritist Center Claudionor de Carvalho (Itabuna, BA, Brazil)
CEI	International Spiritist Council
CELV	Spiritist Center Light and Truth (Marília, SP, Brazil)
DSV	German Spiritist Association
ESDE	Systematic Study of the Spiritist Doctrine
FEB	Spiritist Federation of Brazil
GEEAK	Spiritist Study Group of Allan Kardec (Munich, Germany)
HEAL	Spiritist Hospital André Luiz (Belo Horizonte, MG, Brazil)
HEM	Spiritist Hospital of Marília (SP, Brazil)
IBGE	Brazilian Department of Geography and Statistics
ICD-10	International Statistical Classification of Diseases and Related Health Problems (10th Revision; WHO)
IMF	International Monetary Fund
IRS	Raúl Soares Institute (Belo Horizonte, MG, Brazil)
SUS	Unitary Health System (Brazil)
UNESP	Federal University of São Paulo State
WHO	World Health Organization

Brazilian and Spiritist Expressions

axé	principle of power/energy in *Candomblé*
bom dia	good morning
caboclo/a	Indigenous spirit in *Candomblé* and *Umbanda*
cachaça	liquor made from sugarcane, comparable to rum
cafezinho	small cup of coffee
Candomblé	Afro-Brazilian religion with roots in West Africa (Angola, Benin, Nigeria)
capoeira	popular Brazilian martial art camouflaged as a dance with roots in Angola
captação	Spiritist diagnostic-therapeutic practice with the help of mediums
chakras	centers of energetic transmission between body, spirit, and *perispirit*
Coroados	Indigenous population in the South and South-East of Brazil
disobsession	mediumship practice to guide afflicted and afflicting spirits (obsessors) toward spiritual progress and stop their harmful effect on living people (Braz.: *desobsessão*)
Espiríta/Espiritismo	Spiritist/Spiritism
evangelho no lar	studying Spiritist doctrine at home, with family and friends
evangelization	lecturing/studying Spiritist doctrine (Braz.: *evangelicação*)
favela	shanty-town, poor neighborhood, or suburb of Brazilian cities
feijoada	Brazilian dish of beans and pork, shared with family and friends on Saturdays
fluids/fluidized	a principle of spiritual energy in Spiritism/charged with spiritual energy
fluidoterapia	treating the fluids of a person, including fluid donation by volunteers

fraternal care	psycho-social-spiritual practice of care provided by (often) non-specialized volunteers, based on Spiritist doctrine and mediumship practice (Braz.: *atendimento fraterno*)
gringo	non-Brazilian, foreigner
guia	spiritual guide; benevolent spirit
jeitinho	smartness, amicable short-cut to reach one's aims by bending the rules
karma	spiritual concept of cause and effect throughout several lifetimes
Macumba	black magic, witchcraft; term often used to denigrate Afro-Brazilian religions
malandragem	trickery, lifestyle of petty crime to reach one's aims with smallest effort
mediumship	sensory perception of spirits and practice of spirit communication (Braz.: *mediunidade*)
moradores	inhabitants (here: of a particular ward/psychiatric unit)
nervos	idiom of distress related to "nervousness" and communicating a state of powerlessness and stress through bodily symptoms, particularly among poor and marginalized populations in Brazil
obsession	state of being affected by the spirit (obsessor) of a deceased person seeking revenge or staying attached to the living, thus causing affliction and being afflicted at the same time; comparable to the concept of (negative) possession (Braz.: *obsessão*)
orixá	Afro-Brazilian spiritual entity/god
passe	energetic treatment of the *perispirit*
perispirit	a subtle energetic body that connects the biological body with the immortal spirit
preto/a velho/a	Afro-Brazilian spirit in *Candomblé* and *Umbanda*
ponto	spiritual chant in *Umbanda*
psychography	automatic writing, mediumship practice
reforma intíma	inner reform by studying and living Spiritist doctrine
sala mediúnica	mediumship hall; a place where mediumship is performed
samba	popular Brazilian music and dance style informed by Afro-Brazilian culture
spiritual surgery	Spiritist therapeutic practice of treating the *perispirit* (and thus, body and mind) on a fluidical level; in the past also physical interventions by alleged spirit doctors through their mediums

telenovela	popular Brazilian soap operas
Umbanda	Brazilian religion fusing Afro-Brazilian religion, Spiritism, Indigenous, and Esoteric practices
Vale do Amanhecer	Brazilian religion that fuses *Umbanda*, Spiritism, Millenarism, and New Age practices

Figures

3.1 Front view of the *Hospital Espírita de Marília*
(Photography by HK 2015)   57
3.2 Topography of HEM (Photography by HK 2015)   61
3.3 HEM's "Theater" (Photography by HK 2015)   63
3.4 Front view of the *Centro Espírita Luz e Verdade*
(Photography by HK 2015)   76
3.5 CELV's Lectures Hall (Photography by HK 2015)   81
4.1 HEM's *Sala Mediúnica* (Mediumship Room)
(Photography by HK 2015)   101
5.1 Psychographic Image of Dr. Hermann (Photography
by HK 2016)   132
5.2 Dr. Hermann's Pharmacy (Photography by HK
2016)   132
5.3 Front view of the *Centro Espírita Claudionor de
Carvalho* (Photography by HK 2016)   135
5.4 CECC's Waiting Room (Photography by HK 2016)   137

Chapter 1

Introduction

Diversification of Mental Healthcare

> The contemporary practice of health, despite all scientific processes, presents itself as a fragmented overspecialization. Besides that, it often lacks individual support regarding resources of self-knowledge, wisdom, and (self-)love, which would be the base of health-seeking behavior in the sense of permanent efficacy. The majority of patients wish for anesthesia instead of conscience. It is alright to reduce the effects of their symptoms to avoid unnecessary and unproductive suffering. Still, the educational process which would free the individuals from their ignorance and dependencies is fundamental to the reconstruction process of health and a precaution against the diseases of body and soul.
>
> (Moreira 2013: 23f; translation HK)

Brazilian Spiritist medical doctor Moreira addresses contested realms of healing at the intersection of scientific and spiritual knowledge, postulating holistic approaches toward health, care, and well-being. He acknowledges the passive positionality of patients being diagnosed according to biomedical and/or psychiatric categories and exposed to treatments rather than actively participating in them. In November 2011, I participated in the 14th Spiritist Congress of the Spiritist Federation of Bahia in the convention center of Salvador da Bahia/Brazil. It is a massive complex with an auditorium and several other meeting facilities. The event was organized as a scientific congress with about 50 lectures and workshops, attracting several hundred participants, including psychologists and medical professionals discussing topics such as "The Human Being as Bio-Psycho-Socio-Spiritual," "Psychology centered in Spiritism," and "Mental Health and Spiritism." The keynote was held by Divaldo P. Franco, president of the Brazilian Spiritist Federation FEB and the contemporary flagship of the international Spiritist movement. He was received like a celebrity and welcomed the participants to the "Primacy of the Spirit." After an initial prayer, he lectured on the history and pioneers of Spiritism and related to several international psychologists whose work would verify related approaches, for example, Ian Stevenson (USA). He talked for over an hour without using a script or any other aid, and by the intonation of his voice, it appeared to me that he was in a trance.

DOI: 10.4324/9781032637167-1

Book tables in the foyer presented literature addressing "Depression and Mediumship," "Clinical Mediumship," and "Spiritist Visions of Mental Disturbances," and throughout the four days of this conference, I gained insights into the latter. One aspect that in the aftermath of this event has caught my attention is the idea that "hearing voices" must not necessarily be diagnosed as a psychiatric problem but as a capacity of mediumship that I have decided to refer to as a "sixth sense" in reminiscence of the 1999 Hollywood blockbuster where "seeing dead people" plays a significant role. For over a decade, I have investigated related Brazilian Spiritist practices in (mental) health/care,[1] exploring their embeddedness in global developments and transcultural and -national relationships, strategies for negotiating divergent therapeutic epistemologies and approaches, and performative, sensory, and aesthetic aspects of healing. As a result, I intend to facilitate the comprehension and appreciation of alternate explanatory models of mental health as aligned to specific socio-cultural frames and processes. Moreover, I have been seeking answers to why specific individuals would seek mental healthcare support within spiritual institutions such as Brazilian Spiritism. I conclude that besides the lack of available resources or the more general quest for "holistic methods," it is the aspect of divergent sensory experiences they may cultivate in particular therapeutic settings. Accordingly, I will elaborate on the Aesthetics of Healing as a toolbox to address, describe, analyze, and interpret mental healthcare practices in Spiritism and beyond. I will link the narratives of involved persons to autoethnographic accounts and participant observational ethnographic data that focuses on the phenomenon of voices framing experiences of affliction and recovery: voices of spirits, patients, therapists, supporters, and other beings involved, that is, voices of good sense. I will explore the sensory techniques that enable specific individuals to develop a "sixth sense," the capacity to perceive, communicate, and negotiate the contesting voices of afflicting and sympathetic spirits. It is beyond my scope and expertise to finally define it as "empathy" or "mediumship," but it responds to Moreira's (ibid.) postulate of new approaches in (mental) healthcare that integrate divergent perspectives beyond those of the healthcare professionals, thus providing agency and giving voice to the afflicted (and the afflicting).

Therapeutic Spaces of Brazilian Spiritism

Brazilian culture displays a wide range of structural violence and social inequalities that cannot entirely be related to specific ethnic, economic, or gender affiliations but to a general negotiation of power and impotence where corruption, smartness (*jeitinho*), and trickery (*malandragem*) consti- tute legitimate shortcuts of taking advantage. It results in continuous social competition and marginalization of weak and impotent members of society who are left to be crushed in the system's gears. Public discourse transfers causes of existing inequalities to divergent levels of adaptation to "modernity" as opposed to "tradition," but they result from the lack of political will to improve power relations and social participation. A widespread cynical response to Stefan Zweig's (2007) declaration of Brazil as the "land of the future" is that it will remain so as long as the many challenges of this young democracy remain unresolved.

From this perspective, the investigation of health-seeking behaviors, explanatory models, divergent health accesses, and resources of so-called "alternative" healing practices have become relevant due to a "panorama of health inequalities in Brazil" (Landmann-Szwarcwald & Macinko 2016). Da Glória Cohn (2010) stresses the importance of non-governmental organizations mobilizing civic resources and independent religious institutions framing an increasing pluralization of care. The resulting diversification of (mental) health/care in Brazil intersects with ideological contests on religion, philosophy, politics, and science that produce new medical discourse. Hess (1987) observes a secularization of religious practices as alternative scientific approaches distinct from comparable "Western" developments, and similarly, Teixera and Menezes (2006) report reconfigurations, transformations, and adaptions of spiritual healing practices as ongoing dynamics of religious transition where new approaches arise and even migrate, transgressing boundaries and adapting to global developments. As a result, in Brazil, psychiatric institutions coexist with numerous religious movements specialized in treating emotional, spiritual, and mental distress (Rabelo 1993), e.g., Kardecist Spiritism ("Kardecism").

Aureliano and Cardoso (2015: 275) state that Spiritism rationalized religious beliefs and practices within specific 19th-century contexts in Europe and North America. This dynamic included the (re)articulation of explanatory models regarding mental health and illness in terms of spiritual parameters. Particularly in Brazil, Spiritists have developed specific psychiatric treatments and currently engage in their global distribution. Spiritists regard spirit obsession and mediumship as explanatory models for affliction. Spirit obsession conceptualizes the attachment of the spirit of a deceased human person to an incarnate individual. Divergent from conceptualizations of possession, the spirits do not take over their victims' bodies but may produce harm on an energetic level and thus influence their behavior. The underlying model of a person differs from Cartesian body–mind distinctions propagated in cosmopolitan medicine; it subdivides into a material mortal body and an immaterial, reincarnating, and progressing spirit. These spheres connect through the *perispirit*, an energetic subtle body that comprises experiences and memories of both the body and the spirit and, therefore, includes what we may refer to as the "mind." Therapists perform *passe* for energetical treatment and *disobsession* as a gentle exorcism where mediums facilitate communication with afflicted and afflicting spirits. In both cases, affected individuals must actively work on their spiritual progress by studying Spiritist knowledge (*evangelization*). *Fraternal care* serves as an emergency treatment where volunteers assist people in despair and organize the before-mentioned treatments. Some mediums also perform *spiritual surgeries* that may be defined as "extended" *passe* that treat, from a biomedical and psychiatric perspective, both somatic and mental afflictions through the *perispirit*. All practices are based on the principle of charity, and many Spiritists further engage in food supplies for the poor and other voluntary projects for their and others' spiritual progress.

The impact of Spiritist practice and discourse on health markets outside Brazil so far has only been marginally addressed (cf. Lewgoy 2008; Voss 2011), but the importance for the Brazilian healthcare system is obvious. Overall, religious healing practices such as those provided by Spiritists often substitute the official health sector, particularly in the mental health sector. Throughout the last decades, Brazilian health policy administrators have aimed to close psychiatric hospitals to redirect care to patients' families and communities. However, those have been left alone with the burden of care due to political mismanagement, economic crisis, unemployment, inflation, and decreased social welfare throughout the second decade of the 20th century and under the influence of divergent governmental orientations and health-political programs. Accordingly, diversifying mental healthcare by religiously/spiritually engaged therapeutic practices constitutes an essential anthropological and interdisciplinary exploration focus. So far, several researchers have addressed the pluralistic field of constructions and experiences of (a)normality from different perspectives, including engagement with spiritual agencies. In this regard, Budden (2010) stresses that divergent traditions cannot be understood as independent medical systems but that they intersect and interact, being shaped and transformed by those seeking health. Accordingly, the Brazilian Spiritist movement has developed a unique form of therapeutic diversification in that it provides institutions that combine psychiatric and spiritual knowledge and practice, particularly within Spiritist psychiatric hospitals and so-called Spiritist centers.

My investigation explores the contemporary situation of Brazilian mental healthcare and how Spiritist institutions contribute. Between 2015 and 2017, I implemented 12 months of multi-sited ethnographic field research in Brazil, starting with the *Hospital Espírita de Marília* (HEM, "Spiritist Hospital of Marília"/São Paulo/Brazil)[2] and affiliated Spiritist centers such as the *Centro Espírita Luz e Verdade* (CELV, "Spiritist Center of Light and Truth") and the *Centro Espírita Barsanulfo* (CEB, "Spiritist Center of Barsanulfo"). I regularly participated in Spiritist meetings, workshops, and treatments before I tracked these institutions' translocal networks. For inner-Brazilian comparison, I performed fieldwork at the *Centro Espírita Claudionor de Carvalho* (CECC, "Spiritist Center of Claudionor de Carvalho") in Itabuna/Bahia/Brazil. However, I also followed another spontaneously materializing network to Munich/Germany, where I conducted another 6 months of field research

(2016–2017) to investigate transnational relations and transformations of practices. I perceived this unexpected option as an opportunity to "close the circle" once that Spiritist knowledge and practice root in 19th century Europe, and after over a century, Brazilian immigrants would (re)introduce them. I participated in the activities of the German Spiritist center *Grupo Espírita de Estudos Allan Kardec e.V.* (GEEAK, "Spiritist Study Group of Allan Kardec,") and followed other health-related Spiritist networks inside Germany.

Each setting served as a location for roughly six months of field research, including participant observation and rapport with psychiatrists, healers, patients, and clients, participating in routines and practices. However, the setting in Germany somewhat constituted a "Third Space" as a cultural contact zone between German adepts of New Age spirituality and Brazilian immigrants seeking support in their migration experiences (see Chapter 5). In all settings, I explored the production of therapeutic spaces and embodied healing practices by implementing methods of participant observation, qualitative interviews, media research, and an innovative approach to sensory ethnography that partially even became autoethnographic when I started to reflect on my experiences of mediumship practices (see Chapter 4).

Mental Health at the Intersection of Religion and Medicine

Within medical anthropology, mental healthcare constitutes a distinct research field at the intersection of individual experience, cultural interpretation, and social-political (re)action toward human affliction (Scheper-Hughes & Lock 1987). It implies the investigation of religious/spiritual institutions complementing psychiatric and official health-political approaches (Basu et al. 2017) and their attitude toward "extraordinary conditions" (Jenkins 2015) and "deviant behavior" (Goode 2019). Shorter's (1997) historical account of the psy-sciences reveals how diagnostic and therapeutic practices have developed and contested according to a respective *Zeitgeist* throughout the last centuries. Accordingly, "psychiatry" is a socio-cultural practice within a particular historical, political, economic, and cosmological context and is not a universally valid science of human conditions or appropriate behaviors. On the contrary, Porter (1987) elaborates that psychiatric patients have always acted "rationally" in their terms but in opposition to what a social majority would deem "normal." Foucault (1988a) concludes that in an age of rationalization and modernization, the label "anormal" has served the negotiation and definition of "normality" within a specific socio-cultural frame, that is, European modernity based on rationality deriving from Enlightenment discourse. He concludes that the history of madness and psychiatry is one of power and control, erasing any practice or discourse deemed irrational or deviant from contemporary social norms, values, and, thus, accepted public discourse and behavior.

For the European example, Porter (1987) and Shorter (1997) illustrate that "mad" behavior has always been a topic of concern but has long been related to external causes such as gods, demons, or fate. In medieval times, discourse on deviant behavior referred to religiously informed imaginations on the competition of God, Satan, and their grip on human souls. Individuals who did not correspond to religiously structured patterns of authorized behavior met social exclusion or even physical extinction in the tortures and pyres of the Catholic Inquisition (and later on, the death industry of the German Nazi regime). On the other hand, divergent interpretations of alternate perceptions and behaviors have existed as divine skills (e.g., Hildegard von Bingen, 1098–1179). As divergent as these explanatory models are, they all depict dualistic models of rationality/irrationality and good/evil that have shaped European cosmologies and, already centuries ago, framed future global mental healthcare policies as an authoritarian tool of public sedation, control, and discipline (cf. Foucault 1988a).

Under neo/colonial rule, medical and psychiatric practices and institutions have been established around the world, and until today, representatives of the neuro- and psy-sciences act on a global scale, regardless of cultural diversities and/or singularities regarding explanatory models, concepts of person, or socio-political-economic contexts that frame ideas of self, community, and "appropriate" behavior. This is not to say that in certain circumstances, conventional psychiatric treatment may help some patients in mental, emotional, or spiritual distress, but in this scenario, any discourse or practice that does not apply to European models of coherent behavior is deemed backward and irrational. Once again, the myth of European superiority precipitates claims to control the rest of the world by distributing psychiatric models, categories, and technologies in contemporary Global (Mental) Health policies. Greene et al. (2011) and Baer et al. (2013) elaborate on the historical context that is, colonial medicine serving three interconnected ends: maintenance of racist superiority discourse, implementation of Christian models of "care," and support of European intruders in environments experienced as hostile. Indigenous patients would have to adapt to Christian beliefs and European ways of life to enjoy new forms of treatment. At the same time, policies of "detribalization" and assimilation produced new (mental) health problems and, therefore, new markets of medical "development assistance." Accordingly, the authors criticize biomedicine and biologically oriented psychiatry as monstrous inventions of a global capitalist economy to maintain and control human resources.

Contemporary attempts to integrate local, often religiously/spiritually informed, knowledge with cosmopolitan healthcare exist but produce asymmetries in promoting biomedicine and psychiatry as superior to Indigenous practices (cf. Basu 2009, 2014a). However, members of marginalized classes, ethnicities, and populations continue to navigate within their autochthonous medical systems as popular, comprehensible, and accessible health resources and as a means of resistance against socio-cultural paternalism and control by Global Health institutions and related economic interests (cf. Huizer 1987; Farmer 2005). This attitude coincides with increasing global requests for so-called "traditional" or "holistic" therapeutic approaches that, as "Complementary and Alternative Medicines" (CAM), contest and complement cosmopolitan measures in biomedicine and psychiatry. Accordingly, one task in medical anthropology is to explore divergent agencies and ideologies in therapeutic settings (cf. Kleinman 1988a; Kirmayer 1989a). Kirmayer (2006) attempts to bridge epistemological gaps by invoking a "new cross-cultural psychiatry" as an interdisciplinary approach exploring local and global contexts, their interrelations and mutual influences, social mobilities, and transfers/transformations of mental health-related knowledge and practice. He assumes that there has always been a constant exchange, circulation, mutual transformation, and proliferation of distinct healing practices and interprets the increasing demand for CAM within Western societies as a hybrid integration of apparently antithetic therapeutic practices and discourses (ibid. 2014: 33). Accordingly, the subversive powers of local healing traditions and demands of patients continue to challenge the biomedical hegemony and related political implications.

Religion is a significant category in investigating cultural, social, and individual meanings of mental health and their negotiation alongside contesting approaches (Incayawar et al. 2009; Verhagen et al. 2010). Dynamics of global migration, mobile social worlds, and mass media even reinforce this process. One focus of related research has thus been to investigate conditions of plural and locally co-existing medical and religious traditions, as well as hybrid and globally expanding CAM responding to diversified health-seeking behavior. Inhorn and Wentzell (2012) address the intersection of medicine and religion and especially the importance of religious care practices within public healthcare sectors in different locations. Accordingly, medical anthropologists must focus on the coexistence, interaction, and translation of medical and religious traditions, promoting divergent explanatory models and interventions regarding mental, spiritual, emotional, and/or (psycho)social distress and integrating spiritual agencies and their impact on the constitution of the self. They implement (re)interpretations of affliction as externally caused, providing moral dimensions, alternate concepts of self and person, and related coping strategies. Existing problems in translating cultural concepts from one therapeutic context to another are not reduced to an insufficient Western model of body and mind or divergent socio-cultural categories but also manifest into individual modes of how persons construct and perceive themselves in different settings. Discussing mental health thus means discussing the constitution of the self in interaction with its lifeworld and in coherence with local environments and conceptualizations of biological, moral, and explanatory models of experience (Csordas 2002; Burns Coleman & White 2010).

Epistemological gaps continue to exist, particularly between patients' illness experiences, therapists' disease diagnoses, and socio-political sickness categories. For the case of India, Basu (2014a) raises the example of the Sufi shrine of Mira Datar in Gujarat as an experimental site of cooperation of cosmopolitan psychiatry with religious healing practices. She explores how discourse on possession is contested between religious healers and psychiatrists, labeling it either a result of schizophrenia, and thus an internal distortion of the self, or as sorcery and, therefore, an external attack. Besides elaborating on opposing concepts of mind, body, and self in terms of individual vs. dividual or permeable selves, Basu criticizes the ideological asymmetries between dominant psychiatric and religiously informed ritual healing practices. Related policies would support the medicalization of psycho-social issues and marginalize, if not delegitimize, subaltern approaches. However, most important for our discussion, she interprets mental health-related practices as socially embedded attempts to (re)create a social/spiritual order that does not locate health, illness, and healing in the individual body of a "self" but in its relations to others.

For decades, human–spirit interactions have attracted the attention of medical anthropologists and interdisciplinary colleagues worldwide, delivering divergent interpretations located somewhere between social or psychological functions, often without acknowledging their coincidence. Many share symbolic and performative perspectives focusing on the interaction of the afflicted selves with their environments. It implies the idea of symbolic acts as healing social relations, including spiritual ones. Accordingly, ritual healing practices generate multivocal meanings relating to particular contexts and experiences (Laderman & Roseman 1996), and for the example of Spiritist movements in Latin America, Schmidt (2015, 2016a) elaborates on some relevant aspects: she illustrates how the anthropological discussion of mediumship has imposed categories such as gender, race, class, identity, resistance, hybridization, and performance that would not value the polyphony, heterogeneity, and diversification of the related fields; the anthropological gaze on structures, functions, and meanings would ignore experiences, narratives, and interpretations of the affected.

For the example of Brazil, Schmidt illustrates the experiential factor of spirit mediumship as an altered state of consciousness involving the "training of abilities" (ibid.: 2016a: 38) and opposing psychiatric interpretations of "dissociation" or "multiple personality disorder" (ibid.: 39). Schmidt (2016b), therefore, directs her attention toward the aesthetic involvement of participants. She further states that though, so far, scientific attention has usually been directed toward the mediums, the audience is crucial for the social aspect of these practices, too (ibid.: 438; cf. ibid. 2017). Leonardi and Schmidt (2020) stress the importance of religious narratives and experiences for well-being and argue that spirituality provides meaning, value, and purpose to life in a fundamentally relational context (ibid.: 1f). Resources of spiritual well-being would support self-acceptance, personal growth, purpose in life, and social interaction. From that perspective, spiritual practices complement mental healthcare in transforming self-perception, sense, and relationality (ibid.: 6).

Healing Cooperation

> Surprisingly, despite anthropological and other social research interest in medical pluralism and critiques of biomedicalization, we have paid little attention to the diverse practices of nonbiomedical therapies in different settings, their introduction and incorporation in new settings, differences in clinic practice and practitioner/client engagement, relationships of different practices and professional organizations, the embodiment of different regulatory contexts [...] or the politics shaping the provision of different modalities [...].
>
> (Nissen and Manderson 2013: 3)

Nissen and Manderson point out the necessity of exploring the diversity of therapeutic practices, their interaction, and their transformation due to changing contexts and frames. In my opinion, related research also needs to investigate patterns of cooperation between biomedical and nonbiomedical therapies and how they respond to social, cultural, religious, political, and economic conditions. Current debates in medical anthropology contest strategies toward integrating cosmopolitan medicine and local healing practices (Incayawar et al. 2009). Especially regarding the globally increasing prevalence of psychiatric diagnoses (WHO 2005, 2014), efforts toward incorporating biomedicine and psychiatry with religious and spiritual healing practices to improve the healthcare systems of so-called developing countries are at stake (WHO 2001, 2017). It unleashes controversial debates on the compatibility of alleged traditional cultural/religious and modern scientific/rational approaches to human experience and how religion and spirituality might contribute to mental healthcare (Bhugra 1996; Kleinman 2012).

Therapeutic cooperation of scientific and religious institutions often remains asymmetrical (Basu 2014a) and is dominated by biomedical discourse that fails to convey socio-cultural frames, meanings, and consequences of illness experience, diagnostic and treatment procedures, and their social embedding. This problem accounts not only for the grassroots level of individual therapy but also for the interdisciplinary collaboration of medical anthropologists, psychiatrists, and biomedical practitioners. Therefore, with the example of Spiritist mental healthcare in Brazil, I tend to explore how different actors in the therapeutic fields take this hurdle and what both practitioners and their clients gain from it.

Demarcation lines between divergent medical systems continuously dissolve, and hybrid therapies develop and globally spread. Local traditions transform into "spiritual" or "esoteric" practices on their journey around the world and contribute to an increasing market of "traditional" healthcare and medical pluralism (cf. Baer et al. 2013). Kirmayer's (2006) perspective on the "ironies of globalization" clarifies that healing practices have constantly been exposed to alien influences and, therefore, per se, establish spaces of fluid and permeable fusion, interpenetration, and hybridization.

Implementing concepts such as "religion/spirituality" and "science/rationality" requires delimitation and a definition of how to apply them. Principally perceiving them as oppositions entails the risk of artificial dichotomization and negating existing interrelations. Instead of assuming a general and ongoing contest of two opposed spheres, Knoblauch (2009), at least in the European context, proposes to acknowledge the dynamics of differentiation and de-differentiation of "religious" and "scientific" explanatory models throughout the 19th and 20th centuries. Applying this perspective to the Brazilian case, I am convinced that dynamics took a different direction or may never have been that explicit. Moreover, medical practices have always situated between the lines of scientific discourse and religious values and eventually became a somewhat "religious" sphere themselves, promoting assumed universal (moral) values and assessing "right" and "wrong" behavior (cf. Adams et al. 2011).

Accordingly, by referring to "religious," "spiritual," and "scientific," "biomedical" therapeutic practices, I do not aim at reproducing academically institutionalized boundaries between diverse therapeutic models. These concepts are only tools to locate medical procedures within a continuum of different ways of integrating the agency of "spiritual beings" or promoting mechanistic perspectives on the human body and how far they integrate socio-cultural aspects. Regarding the ongoing anthropological debate on the differentiation of "religion" and "spirituality" (van Niekerk 2018; Rocha 2017), I do not recognize any epistemological value of distinguishing "institutional" and "individual" practices and subsequently emanating academic categories but instead decide to take into consideration the self-denomination of involved agents: most Spiritists acknowledge the religious traits of their engagement but would rather refer to it as "spiritual-scientific." However, for clarification, I use the term "religion" for institutionalized and transcendental-oriented cultural practices and symbolic systems, whereas I refer to "spirituality" as any form of interaction with spiritual agencies. As both perspectives can hold for Kardecist Spiritism, I will refer to it as a "religious/spiritual" approach without contesting its alleged "scientific" character: Kardecism promotes a "rational" system of spiritual knowledge (see Chapter 2) that may confuse "Western" natural scientists but does not lack any inner logic. Kardecists align with positivist methods of verification and evaluation, particularly when it comes to experiences of health, illness, and healing.

Medical anthropologists have applied the versatile space of coexistence, interaction, and intersection of therapeutic practices to theoretical models such as "medical pluralism," "multiple medical realities" (Johannessen & Lázár 2006), "medical diversity" (Parkin 2013), "medical landscapes" (Hsu 2008a), or "medicoscapes" (Hörbst & Wolf 2014). However, according to Schubert and Voss (2018: 12), most contributions miss the complexity of healing practices involving a wide range of human and non-human actors. Moreover, many would fail in conceiving prominent issues of empowerment or emancipation of patients and their negotiation of popular resources with the specialized knowledge of diverse healers. Therefore, healing cooperation practices do not automatically implement proactive efforts of the therapists' mutual support but derive from the patients' will.

Considering the globally increasing numbers of psychiatric diagnoses and complaints about insufficient therapy resources (WHO 2014, 2017), local treatment structures must be further investigated. A critical analysis implies a closer look at actual practices of healing cooperation and their transformation within translocal networks of healing in terms of exploring interactions, entanglements, and dynamics of therapeutic agencies (Krause et al. 2012: 15f). Csordas (2017) vividly narrates a case of healing cooperation among academically trained mental health professionals and native spiritual healers within a Navajo reservation in the USA. Subsequently, establishing a local, community-based adolescent therapeutic unit aims to integrate psychiatric approaches with Indigenous spiritual concepts and practices and, on a long scale, enhances sustained therapy success. As a supplement to pharmaceutical and conversation-based psychotherapeutic interventions, Csordas highlights his observations of a "traditional" sweat lodge where young patients, even though (or maybe due to) lacking affiliation with Navajo cosmological and spiritual knowledge systems and practices, encounter and interact with "disturbing spirits." This process might not "cure" in terms of restoring health but "heal" in the sense of developing coping strategies aligned with external social and spiritual forces (ibid.: 132f; cf. Waldram 2013). Inferentially, local religious and psychiatric explanatory models can complement, inspire each other, and fuse into new practices of cooperation to restore mental health by spiritual transformation. Mediumship practices are particularly interesting here as they integrate spiritual and social aspects of affliction in terms of embodied learning processes toward altered perceptions and experiences of self and social relations, resulting in a particular sense of health and healing.

Aesthetics of Healing

Medical anthropologists increasingly explore the sensory production of therapeutic settings, stressing the relevance of bodily experience as crucial for the health-seeking behavior of patients (Desjarlais 1992; Halliburton 2009; Alex 2018). Similarly, anthropologists of religion address the "aesthetic" quality of religious experience (Münster 2001; Traut & Wilke 2015). Linking these approaches with an emphasis on mental health, my analysis focuses on how Spiritist spaces of healing mental, spiritual, and/or affective afflictions are created by "working with the senses." From a phenomenological perspective (Desjarlais & Throop 2011), the concepts of embodiment (Csordas 1990) and the mindful body (Scheper-Hughes & Lock 1987) extrapolate the dichotomy of body and mind within "Western" cosmologies and scientific approaches as grounded in a fundamental distinction between rationality and emotion, or, in other words, cognitive and sensory perception. Current research in the cultural and social sciences transcends this dichotomy with an extended focus on social and cultural foundations of aesthetics and sensory experience. Accordingly, an increasingly influential anthropology of the senses has produced innovative approaches, concepts, and tools of particular value in medical, religious, and media anthropology: they imply the idea of the human sensorium as socially and culturally produced and constructed. Howes (2005), for example, regards the senses as media that produce and represent socio-cultural meaning to medical or spiritual phenomena. He focuses on the social implications and intersubjective interactions construed by sensory perception and attachment (cf. Chau 2008; Hsu 2008b; Vannini et al. 2012). Hinton et al. (2008) highlight such a focus on the senses in medical anthropology as essential for exploring transformative experiences of healing and health-seeking behavior in diversified therapeutic markets. It implies questioning clinical and cosmological constructions of normal and abnormal sensory experience: whereas psychiatrists may declare visual or auditory perceptions not shared by others as "hallucinations" and thus symptoms of a severe psychosis/schizophrenia (McCarthy-Jones 2012), in religious-spiritual contexts, they may also be interpreted as special skills, e.g., mediumship. Place-making is another aspect of how spaces of healing experience, belonging, identification, and self-transformation are produced. Spaces shape bodies, and bodies create spaces through movement, experience, and interaction (Rodaway 1994). Howes (2005: 7) refers to it as emplacement, a complex network of sensory experiences and interactions, or, in other words, specific body–mind environments.

To investigate these aspects of mental healthcare, I suggest (re)introducing the concept of "Aesthetics of Healing" as a methodological tool for exploring body/mind environments in therapeutic spaces. The terms "aesthetics" and "healing" are critical concepts, as they are highly contested between and within several academic disciplines and orientations. However, in their combination, I consider them fruitful for describing, analyzing, and interpreting therapeutic practices. The concept of aesthetics covers distinct aspects and meanings. Current public and academic discourse often relates to the philosophical interpretation of human expression and its evaluation in artistic and/or moral terms (Kutschera 1988; Sharman 1997). However, considering the original meaning of the ancient Greek word *aísthēsis*, the concept relates to sensory perception as delimited from rational-cognitive processes (Münster 2001). It refers to affective arrangements (Slaby et al. 2017), including symbols, performative elements, media, perception manipulation, and particular body schemes and techniques. As a theoretical tool, the concept of aesthetics thus delimits from culture-bound and philosophical evaluations of human practice and instead refers to intersections of bodily/sensory perceptions and actions with cognitive processes of moral education and evaluation as socio-cultural systems of meaning (Münster 2001: 30f). Nichter (2008), in this regard, argues for a sensorial engaged medical anthropology to study healthcare-seeking and -provision trajectories. He postulates the investigation of cultural responses to the perceptual output of sense modalities (e.g., touch, taste, smell, sight, and sound) as well as sensations (e.g., dizziness, shortness of breath, chest and heart pain, indigestion, states of hot and cold, or shifts in "energy") that conjoin mental and/or emotional states with physical conditions. He wonders how sensations trigger embodied memories and how therapeutic environments may affect these.

Medical anthropologists have often used the concept of "healing" as opposed to "curing" (Strathern & Stewart 1999). This epistemological gap risks imposing dichotomies ontologically derived within Western scientific institutions upon other health knowledge systems (Waldram 2000, 2013). The consequence is an epistemological distinction between "curing" as a primarily biological process emphasizing the removal of a pathological or restoration of a physical state, whereas "healing" refers to broader psychosocial processes regarding the transformation of affective, social, and spiritual dimensions. However, Waldram clarifies that any medical system is a cultural system that engages in both healing and curing (ibid. 2000: 605f). Whereas curing more likely refers to a measurable reduction, reversion, or prevention of specific physiological parameters, healing would connect with personal and subjective experiences involving a reconciliation of meaning and a perception of the "wholeness" as a person. Egnew (2005) defines healing as a personal experience of transcending suffering (ibid.: 255); it may or may not entail curing and involves the perception of positive qualitative changes in the condition of the afflicted and their environment (Waldram 2000: 607).

Accordingly, I conceptualize curing as just one aspect of healing. The terms do not represent opposed ideas or approaches; quite the opposite, healing is paramount to curing: healing addresses any practice of care, regardless of its restorative and/or transformational qualities. With these premises, investigating the Aesthetics of Healing implicates exploring sensory aspects of care that transgress health professionals' limited perspectives on effectiveness and the restoration of bodily states toward integrating patients into the healing experience and supporting their agency. It means investigating "somatic modes of attention" (Csordas 1993) as elaborated ways of attending to and with one's body in interactional healing encounters. In this regard, practices of hospital mimicry,[3] that is, symbolically imitating biomedical practices to meet the expectations of patients, only constitute one aspect in line with Laderman and Roseman (1996), who state that "[a]ll medical and healing encounters are performances as much as technical acts" (ibid.: 1).

The concept of Aesthetics of Healing was first introduced by Bruce Kapferer (1983) in his investigation of Singhalese exorcist practices, where he further develops Turner's (1968a,b) performative approach to symbolic healing by integrating reflections on cognitive meanings of symbols and their sensory communication that would not just serve the healing experience of a single person but the reconfiguration of an entire social environment. As a core quality of healing practices, he identifies "[s]ound, song, smell, dance, and drama [that] combine into what can only be described as a marvelous spectacle which engages all the senses" (Kapferer 1983: 177). Kapferer describes healing rituals as complex compositions of aesthetic forms, modes, and structures that shape experiences and transform (self-)perceptions of participants: he elaborates on the quality of ritual performance as a mode of metacommentary to illustrate, criticize, and negotiate social implications of affliction and well-being. However, as much as social dynamics and cultural context are essential for comprehending healing practices, we must try to understand what occurs within individuals, their feelings, experiences, and needs throughout healing. Dox (2016) stresses her point of view that performances of healing and spirituality do not merely represent something but that practitioners have to be taken seriously by their terms and sensed experience. She does not take spirituality as a symbolic representation but as a kind of bodily engagement, considering the relationship between corporeal sensation, perception, rational thought, and the material world. She directs herself to the question of what kind of (internal) sense of Self is cultivated in spiritual practices and postulates research strategies turning to the body as the primary source of knowledge – for both the researched and researchers. Concluding her critique of representational, symbolical, cognitive, and, therefore, psychological approaches to spiritual healing practices, Dox states:

> The performance paradigm makes the self a subject position and embeds the possibility of an agential self into a critique of the individual, autonomous Western subject. Thus, the paradigm has emphasized how people embody culturally proscribed identities marked by race, class, gender, (dis) ability, and sexuality to read the self as a site of hybrid cultural and social identities operated upon by legislated social norms. In this mode of thinking, there is no concept of the self without a body

situated in and marked by culture. This paradigm emphasizes that there is no essential or authentic self, despite practitioners' assertions of the opposite.

(Dox 2016: 132)

The aspect of how notions of "authentic Selves" are (re)produced in Spiritist practices and how they relate to "Others" will be of central interest in Chapter 4. The process of "othering" includes negotiating socio-cultural impacts and perceptions but goes beyond. Bell (1992) has already criticized the "performative as solely representational" approach by postulating to rethink alleged oppositions between "thought" and "action" in ritual activities. Instead of interpreting practices as paradigmatic acts or attempts of the restoration of social frames and relations, she suggests focusing on dynamics of embodiment to not reduce perception to cognitive *or* sensory aspects of ritual interaction but on *how* rituals and bodies shape each other in the sense of multidirectional influences (Bell 2006). It has been in particular Edith Turner (1992, 2004, 2012) whose approaches have been crucial in investigating "experience in ritual" and its impact on religious healing. Related cultural practices, therefore, are not to be referred to as a cultural text or fixed social structure but appear to address dialectic negotiations within delimited discursive frames. Her approach addresses the interconnections of environment and Self in relating external forms and contents to internal realms of attachment, affection, experience, expectation, images, ideas, impressions, thoughts, and wishes. With such a perspective, we may acknowledge that "Selves" do not embody experience in terms of passive participation but active engagement in healing practices. This aspect of agency, of active participation and experienced practice, its perception, reflection, and reaction to these experiences is of particular interest when exploring the human body and its sensorium in the context of Spiritist mental healthcare. Applying the toolbox of the Aesthetics of Healing, we must examine how internal and external factors connect and interrelate in the course of healing (cf. Sayers 2004).

Contemporary debates often refer to Csordas and his implementation of "embodiment as a paradigm in [medical] anthropology" (ibid. 1990). One of his central insights is that perception and practice are interrelated processes of negotiating passively embodied social structures and actively structuring experiences within a nexus of collective customs and personal needs. In this context, "attention" is a concept of particular interest as it applies to "mindful" processes of bodily, cognitive, and sensory dedication to Self and Others: it denominates dynamics where humans dedicate their bodies as perceptional and communicating agencies within frameworks of culturally shaped practices of bodily interaction and care in the presence of others. To discuss the Aesthetics of Healing thus also means relating to processes of skill and its scaling. Ingold (2013) may serve as a reference point here once he describes enskillment as an education of attention. He refers to skill as a space of creative growth (ibid.: 2000) and argues that skill does not simply represent knowledge but instead displays sensory engagement and acquisition as a creative practice to link the body to its environment, not in terms of a passively incorporated habitus but as a transformative agency (cf. Bourdieu 1977; Giddens 1979). Ingold (2001) thus suggests exploring shared meanings and evaluations of practices regarding their purposefulness and functionality within particular environments and their underlying rules, principles, and negotiations.

These perspectives take further the task of a performative turn within the social and cultural sciences by not only relating to symbolic practices and social aspects but also integrating the individuals' experiences and positioning into the analysis of spiritual healing practices. Accordingly, Bull and Mitchell (2015) outline the potential of combining neuro-anthropology, cognitive anthropology, performance studies, and the anthropology of the senses to develop a new understanding of health-related transmissions in religious, spiritual, and ritual practices (ibid.: 1). Neuro-anthropology would provide insights into biological factors of socio-cultural engagement and, therefore, into "what happens inside the person" (ibid.: 5) and how sensory techniques shape the (re)organization of perception (cf. Howes 2015: 154f).

This is where "culture" enters the stage: specific sensory experiences might be triggered, perceived, interpreted, and evaluated differently among distinct socio-cultural practices (Classen 1993; Howes 2003; Seligman et al. 2016). Applying Nichter's (2008) appreciation of the sensory in medical anthropology, I consider healing a manipulation and reorganization of sensory perception and attention. I do not discuss efficacy once it would be beyond my scope and expertise, but for the sake of understanding how Spiritist practices of mental healthcare affect people and attract them to engage, I will outline sensory aspects of treatment (see Chapters 3–5). I take it with Howes (2009), who discusses religious-spiritual practices as capacities to cultivate a "sixth sense" to (re)organize and (re)frame experiences of "Self" and "Other." However, whereas he refers to experiences and practices of mediumship as "extra-sensory" perception (ibid.: 6f), I am convinced there is no perception without sensory engagement. Instead, I suggest treating mediumship and spirit–human interaction phenomena as divergent sensory experiences that link external stimuli with some "inner sense" that can be triggered, trained, and cultivated.

Several contemporary popular health practices like Yoga, meditation, and mindfulness training are designed to focus on multiple bodily sensations and are increasingly adopted in psychotherapeutic settings. Originally deriving from Asian religious-spiritual contexts, they cultivate particular qualities of attention and awareness grounded in silence, stillness, and self-inquiry. Systematic training and cultivation of sensory engagement, as well as learning to train the perception of internal stimuli (interoception), aim at reflecting on experiences of inadequate or disturbed self-awareness as causes for afflictions. Paying attention to oneself, therefore, may initiate a transformation of self-perception and, thus, recovery of various disturbances (Farb et al. 2015; Kabat-Zinn 2003; Kirmayer 2015). I argue that similar dynamics are at stake for the example of Brazilian Spiritist mental healthcare. As I will elaborate in Chapter 4, mediumship and other therapeutic practices cultivate interoceptive processes toward a "sixth sense" where the "voices" of spirits and other participants play a significant role.

Kardecism in Brazil is an example of healing cooperation between mental health professionals and religious/spiritual experts. By focusing on its Aesthetics of Healing, I will outline how mental healthcare links to educational processes of attention toward "Self" and "Other." These aesthetic trajectories will further suggest innovative perspectives on the 21st-century mental healthcare system in Brazil and beyond.

Translocal Relations

Terms of cultural engagement, whether antagonistic or affiliative, are produced performatively. The representation of difference must not be hastily read as the reflection of pre-given ethnic or cultural traits set in the fixed tablet of tradition. The social articulation of difference, from the minority perspective, is a complex, ongoing negotiation that seeks to authorize cultural hybridizations that emerge in moments of historical transformation. [...] The borderline engagements of cultural difference may as often be consensual as conflictual; they may confound our definitions of tradition and modernity [...].

(Bhabha 1994: 3)

Bhabha's (1994) contribution to a "global ethnography" (cf. Brickell & Datta 2011) implies that in the context of postcolonial socio-cultural entanglements, practices, and knowledge do not simply transfer from one space to another but interact, intersect, and intermingle. He refers to this space of negotiation and hybridization as a "Third Space" that contradicts the notion of a unilinear "modernization" distributed to the world by an alleged "European" superiority (cf. Eisenstadt 2017). On the contrary, Bhabha promotes a perspective describing "alternative modernities" (cf. Gaonkar 2001) as local processes of adaption and adaptation. Accordingly, "modern" customs do not oppose "traditional" ones but derive from an ongoing and continuous transformation of practices, that is, culture as a dynamic process of exchange, communication, negotiation, and appropriation. Especially when turning from the frame of autonomous small-scale societies or local dynamics to contexts of migration, cultural exchange, and translocal relationships, human interaction diversifies due to multiple factors (individual, economic, political, socio-cultural, religious, etc.). In this regard, it is a fundamental observation that migrants often do not become "immigrants" in terms of assimilating to another social structure but appear as "transmigrants" who negotiate varieties of practice and knowledge (Schiller et al. 1995). Accordingly, Machleidt (2013) does not interpret migration as a spatial journey but as a transformation of self and personhood regarding the (re)creation of identity. He claims that expectations often remain unfulfilled due to political restrictions and social practices of exclusion, and many migrants worldwide would seek relief in so-called parallel societies. Those would provide social support, relief of afflicting experiences, and space for (re)orientation in an environment perceived as hostile and exclusive. Networks of care (cf. Thiesbonenkamp-Maag 2014) would mitigate experiences of isolation and discrimination and, therefore, minimize the danger of mental health issues of people being "betwixt and between" (Machleidt 2013: 17f; cf. Turner 1968a). Religious and spiritual practices would create Third Spaces between "here" and "there" that facilitate gradual detachment from the former and adaption to new contexts. They alleviate traumatic experiences of lacking a sense of belonging, help to make sense of experiences, and support the development of agency (ibid.: 98f).

Eichler (2008) stresses the importance of transnational networks as health resources for migrants to negotiate opposing explanatory models and substitute access restrictions to official healthcare services due to legal implications (cf. Huschke 2013). She highlights some salutogenic qualities of those networks and their ability to minimize health risks related to psycho-social acculturation stress. However, in contrast to Machleidt, who eventually locates the skill of successful integration in transcultural psychotherapeutic interventions, Eichler (2008: 31f) argues that it is the location in transnational spaces that implies extraordinary health-related competencies due to their intersection with different socio-cultural practices, and their expertise in creating hybrid and cooperative spaces of (self)-care. Stelzig-Willutzki (2012), in this regard, focuses on the situation of Brazilian women in Germany and the importance of comparable networks for their well-being as often the only resource of social support and care, regardless of the heterogeneity of this social group (ibid.: 153). As Gruner-Domić (2005) generally states for Latin American immigrants in Germany, Stelzig-Willutzki (2012: 229) observes a continuous identification with Brazil as the land of origin and, therefore, ongoing maintenance of translocal networks and relationships (ibid.: 159). However, not only do transmigrants seek support in religious-spiritual practices of their respective cultural origin, but also an increasing number of German patients apply to these spiritual sources of well-being and integrate them into their health-seeking behavior. Duncan (2012) has already discussed what Spiritist centers offer outside of Brazil, and I will elaborate on the transnational and -cultural implications of Kardecism in Chapters 2 and 5, particularly concerning an increasing number of German patients looking for so-called Complementary and Alternative Medicines (CAM) and starting to engage with Spiritism (cf. Voss 2011). Before doing so, I will compare translocal relations of Spiritism *in* Brazil to explore how (healing) practices are transferred and transformed within and between divergent localities.

Jean and John Comaroff (2012) stress the multidirectionality of social practices traveling between the Global South and North, but their argument assumes that impulses from the former are to be interpreted as reactions to the latter. Vertovec and Cohen (2002) contradict this perspective, stressing the diversity and divergences of causes, aims, implementations, and experiences of transnational dynamics. Furthermore, Gottowik (2010) critically questions concepts of transnationality or transculturality in the social sciences as categories that divide nations, cultures, or religions into strictly separate units. Instead of exclusively focusing on national frames, he implements a "translocal" perspective on the mobility of actors, practices, and ideas within and between spaces. Many borders (and their transgression) exist inside and outside the construct of the nation-state in political, religious, social, and economic terms, and their investigation must consider the spatial considerations of the actors themselves (ibid.: 180f). Transnationality, then, is nothing else than a subcategory of a translocal approach, which further diversifies into notions of locality (as homeland or place of origin/belonging) and location (as a space of being/acting) (ibid.: 181). Accordingly, the paradigm of translocality promises a more differentiated investigation of practices, relations, and networks in/between different spaces apart from national categories. Brickell and Datta (2011: 3) argue that while transnationalism would focus on deterritorialized social networks and (economic) exchanges, translocality takes an agency-oriented approach to individual experiences that deliberately confuses the boundaries of the local to capture the increasingly complicated nature of spatial processes and identities as both place-based and mobile. It does not reduce to shared social relations of local histories, experiences, and relations but connects to broader geographical processes. For the scientific study of religions, Bretfeld (2012: 423) suggests perceiving history as a continuous global interaction, flow, entanglement, and network. From this perspective, religion is not an ahistorical entity but a set of practices that permanently transform, re-locate, and intersect. In his discussion of the modalities of transnational transcendence, Csordas (2009) accordingly highlights the fact that modalities of religious intersubjectivity are both transcending cultural boundaries and forging new ones (ibid.: 1). Even though these modalities are explicitly religious, "they are immersed in the political and economic, social and cultural, institutional and ideological" (ibid.). He perceives the "globalization of religion" as a multidirectional flow of practices and meanings with a particular network character (ibid.: 2f).

These considerations also apply to health-related aspects: various researchers have investigated the global circulation of local healing practices (Zanini et al. 2013; Beaudevin & Pordié 2016) and distinct models of healing cooperation in specific contexts. Moreover, the coexistence, interaction, and translation of religious-therapeutic practices in different localities constitute an increasing area of research. Geographies of religious-spiritual healing practices (cf. Barnes 2011) manifest in so-called therapeutic markets (Hüwelmeier & Krause 2010; Klinkhammer & Tolksdorf 2015). They do not merely present divergent therapy models that integrate spiritual agencies into the constitution of self but (re)interpret affliction in specific spatial and temporal terms. Moral dimensions, concepts of personhood, and spiritual approaches to coping with trauma intersect and sometimes complement, substitute, or oppose dominant cosmopolitan medicine *and* local customs, thus bearing conflict potential. It is valid for both local and translocal contexts and their global circulation (Bell et al. 2018) that emerges not only from migration but also from the health-seeking behavior of patients who experience public systems of care as insufficient (Cohen 2017). It particularly applies to the mental healthcare sector with its increasing economization and the implied pathologization and medicalization of deviant behavior (cf. Kohrt & Mendenhall 2015). Controversies manifest in health-related human rights agendas (Jain & Orr 2016), community-based care (Pols 2016), and "counter-clinics," which constitute spaces of well-being with alternative methods of treatment (Davis 2018). It includes the question of how far the diversified, somehow contrary, but also interconnected usages of concepts addressing "intra-/inter-/trans-local/-national/-cultural" realms serve as proper measurements of socio-cultural practices and their transformation. Anthropologists participate in practices, describe, and analyze them, but they cannot claim to observe differences and transformations; this already implies an act of interpretation due to their categories of observation and comparison.

Being aware of these implications and pitfalls, my comparison of different spaces of (Brazilian) Spiritist (mental) healthcare does not intend to generate general allegations on transforming practices in different settings but to outline certain developments in specific, interconnected localities within a delimited space-time context. These interconnections developed rather by coincidence than providence, and I followed them without considering them representative of any "general" Spiritist practices or their transformation. I introduce them as exemplary for dynamics I observed on a translocal level, applying categories of comparison I developed in the previous chapters, particularly Healing Cooperation and Aesthetics of Healing. I will explore healing spaces and practices within the translocal networks of Brazilian Spiritism.

Making Sense

Wondering about "[w]hat counts as data," Tanya Luhrmann (2010: 212) illustrates a gap between practices of ethnographic description and anthropological interpretation that also accounts for spirit–human relations: as researchers and authors, we describe certain settings and interpret them in terms of theoretical models, e.g., as performance, altered states of consciousness, and saluto- or pathogenic experiences. Interviews with mediums may provide some insight into their experiences, but those remain second- or third-hand accounts. This observation raises the question of how we might be able not merely to study forms but also the contents of practices.

I still recount my first mediumship session, accompanied by my wife, who used to frequent *Umbanda* but has never engaged in mediumship practices. Throughout this *disobsession* event, *obsessors* (afflicting spirits of deceased people) and *guias* (spiritual guides different from those in *Candomblé* or *Umbanda*) were incorporated by participating mediums. Contrary to general customs, that night, the Indigenous *caboclo* spirit of Jurema, usually worshiped in *Umbanda*, introduced herself as my *guia*, blessing my "significant" endeavor. She intended to sing a *ponto* (*Umbanda* chant) to support me spiritually but was not allowed to as the supervisor of this meeting argued that "this is not the right space for it." I later learned that her medium, an elderly lady, had previously engaged with *Umbanda* but now sought "deeper knowledge" here. Accordingly, I could have taken this episode as a performative expression of the demarcations Kardecists like to draw between their practices and alleged "lower Spiritisms" (see Chapter 2) if it was not for two observations: before, throughout, and still after this incident, my wife had bodily compulsions typical for spirit incorporations in *Umbanda*. She had never been in this town before and had rarely engaged with Kardecism before, but ever since that day, she would have similar reactions in some *Umbanda* centers we visited. To a lesser degree, the same is true for me, and this is my second observation: for many years, I have been fascinated by Brazilian *caboclo* spirits and *orixás* (Afro-Brazilian spiritual entities) and even envisioned some of them after hours of drumming, singing, and dancing. However, I was always aware of what I was *supposed* to perceive once events were dedicated to certain entities, with their public illustrations shaping my imagination. This time, I did not know what to expect at all, but still, my body was shaking and shivering. I experienced a soothing feeling of happiness, calmness, and relaxation. I had hardly ever felt this before but repeatedly would do so again throughout my field research (see Chapter 4).

Regarding spirit mediumship practices in therapy, Bowie (2016) speaks of insider/outsider perspectives and the negotiation of blurred boundaries. She outlines the "mental gymnastics" researchers have to practice at the intersection of "methodological agnosticism," that is, ignoring the researcher's experience for the sake of some alleged objective interpretation devoid of bias (ibid.: 2). However, my methodology envisions the experimental approach of an experience-near and multimodal medical anthropology (cf. Wikan 1991; Pink 2011; Cartwright & Crowder 2017). Luhrmann (2010), in this regard, mentions "non-cognitive modes of learning" as bodily, emotional, or imaginal ways of knowing. These modes evoke sudden and flashing experiences as they often illuminate the limits of cognitive learning by showing how "raw" emotive moments can be informative. This non-cognitive experience is described as visceral, emotional, and highly unpredictable. As anthropologists, we can thus learn through practice in terms of "deep participation" that addresses "the ways of approaching people's lifeworlds and inner scapes, especially when dealing with other intangible worlds and selves involved in their spiritual practices" (Pierini & Groisman 2016: 1).

Pink (2009) addresses the realm of sensory practice and experience as both a research field and a methodological approach in terms of reflecting and rethinking our participatory research techniques (ibid.: 8f) toward what she calls "embodied knowing" (ibid.: 15). Accordingly, experience relates to our environment and our strategies to integrate with it in social, behavioral, emotional, sensory *and* cognitive terms. Our attempts to deduct structures and impose categories are constantly disturbed by particular configurations and performative interactions that are bodily experienced (ibid.: 33). Therefore, we should not only investigate how our research partners learn through sensory embodied experiences and memories but also how we do so (ibid.: 34). I have integrated this approach into my methodology, particularly in the mediumship context. I explore the sensory qualities of diagnostic and therapeutic practices and also reflect on my engagement in the context of participant observation as a means of data collection and handling my subjective experiences.

As the classical method of ethnography, participant observation transforms into more insightful observing participation when carried out with care, empathy, and attention. It becomes a phenomenological approach that integrates sensory, emotional, and cognitive aspects of experience. Further developing Geertz's (1973) approach of thick description, Spittler (2001) promotes the method of thick participation as a radicalized form of data collection that implies apprenticeship and practice, natural conversation and observation, lived experience, and sensuous research that integrates the researcher's experience and sensory perception (cf. Pink 2009). Without going native, I felt pretty integrated in most settings, and I was able to verify my perceptions and interpretations by discussing them with my interlocutors. However, developing comparable parameters and categories in such diverse and divergent environments as healthcare institutions was a challenge. As van der Geest and Finkler (2004) illustrate in their discussion on hospital ethnography, hospitals are not identical clones of a global biomedical model but take on different forms in different cultures and societies. They become domains where core values and beliefs of culture come into view and thus reflect and reinforce dominant social and cultural processes in terms of negotiation and (re)configuration of experience, normality, selfhood, and belonging. Accordingly, Long et al. (2008) stress the multiple meanings of hospitals as liminal spaces with religious, social, economic, political, and perceptional aspects.

A red thread of my investigation in all settings is to understand and compare procedures of "making the other" (cf. van Dongen 2004) in Spiritist psychiatric hospitals and community centers in Brazil and Germany, where Brazilian immigrants and German affiliates would interact. How would they establish and refer to the Other, and how would I, as an anthropologist, develop new perspectives on it by interaction and adaption? Further, how should I refer to my personal experiences? Van Dongen illustrates in one of her field note anecdotes the request of a patient: "What are you writing? Are you writing down your findings? Fine! But do write about *me*! (a woman from the hospital)" (ibid.: 279). I had similar experiences, and accordingly, I follow van Dongen's postulate to listen to alternative rationalities, realities, and experiences beyond cognitive anthropological categories. I implemented narrative and semi-structured interview techniques alongside expert interviews and focused conversations to keep the spectrum of possible interview partners as wide as possible. They included patients, therapists, participants, and outsiders. Due to the friendly openness of Brazilian Spiritists and their mutual interest in having their practices explored scientifically, I conducted over 50 narrative interviews. Most of these interviews have been recorded, and I anonymized them when my research partners requested. However, most have insisted on appearing with their real name; those who did not are anonymized without being marked. I also recorded conversations with patients and mediumship sessions. I did so with the agreement of the involved persons (including spirits). However, patients and other vulnerable individuals will appear anonymized again without being specifically marked. Imagined names do not correspond to any other people I met in the field, and I am convinced that this way, I can best stick to my ethical responsibility once it remains unclear which research partners appear with their real or fantasy names.

Even though mediumship appears to be central to Spiritism, it does not exist apart from other practices and is of even less relevance in the healing experiences of patients. To entirely grasp Spiritist approaches to mental health, we must step back for approximately 200 years to inquire about early developments in Europe and translocal relations that will take us to Brazil and, in the 21st century, finally back to Germany. Chapter 2 introduces the history of Spiritism as parallel to the ascension of the psychiatric discipline in 19th-century Europe and 20th-century Brazil. A review of interdisciplinary accounts explores correlations between psychiatry and Spiritism in Brazil and outlines contemporary developments in healthcare. Central concepts, practices, and their transformation are explored and related to contested political, economic, and socio-cultural developments. Divergent interpretations and evaluations of Spiritist practices illuminate their importance for the Brazilian context and address translocal aspects that will again be of particular interest in Chapter 5. Chapter 3 introduces the research site of Marília with its divergent Spiritist mental healthcare resources. It presents rich ethnographic data on healing cooperation between Spiritists and mental healthcare professionals and provides a closer gaze at actual practices and specific explanatory models that shape disease categories, illness experiences, and related social implications, not being static but dynamic and flexible within given individual contexts and social situations. Chapter 4 is dedicated to social and aesthetic fabrications of therapeutic spaces and aligns with phenomenological approaches addressing the question of sensory experience and embodied healing. Partly based on autoethnographic data, the argument contributes to the discussion of the Aesthetics of Healing as a theoretical tool to explore the particularities of Brazilian Spiritist mental healthcare but also to provide new perspectives for medical anthropology in general. Considering translocal trajectories and transformations of Spiritist practices, Chapter 5 investigates aspects of divergent implementation, scaling, and adaptation of Spiritist healing practices to respective contexts and environments in Brazil and abroad. Spiritist approaches to mental healthcare in Brazil are already bifurcated due to regional and ideological differences. Based on the hypothesis that they would even more so in transcultural contexts, the chapter compares therapeutic spaces of Spiritism in Brazil and Germany and how participants contest, negotiate, and transform ideas and practices according to their subjective scopes, needs, and experiences. Chapter 6 summarizes my insights regarding the translocal dynamics of the diversification of mental healthcare at the intersection of psychiatry and religion with the example of Brazilian Spiritist mental healthcare.

Notes

1   I use brackets and slashes to facilitate the discussion of interrelated but still divergent aspects: (mental) health/care indicates that I address health, mental health, healthcare, and mental healthcare. Whereas the differentiation between health and healthcare is quite apparent, somatic and mental health cannot be separated as concepts because they intersect. Furthermore, with the example of Brazilian Spiritism, these delimitations do not make any sense because the Cartesian body–mind dualism is substituted by a more complex model of spirit-*perispirit*-body with the "mind" located in the interaction of these spheres.
2   All institutions and many research participants insisted on me not anonymizing them as they interpreted my research as a means of communicating their perspectives. For those who wanted to be anonymized, I will change their names without marking them. I am convinced this is the most ethical way to respect my interlocutors' wishes and expectations.
3   I do not use this term as a pejorative term. I conceptualize hospital mimicry as performative practices that sometimes support the patient's sense of being treated (see Chapter 5).

Chapter 2

Spiritism and Mental Health

In October 2016, I attended a conference on mediumship and (mental) health/care in Bad Honneff, Germany. The *PsychoMedizin Kongress* ("Psycho-Medicine Congress") attracted about a hundred persons, including some Brazilian immigrants and guest speakers, but mainly German participants with divergent backgrounds in New Age movements, anthroposophical medicine, quantum medicine, holistic medicine, psychotherapy, and biomedicine. The foci of lectures were on reincarnation and mediumistic healing, including studies by US-American Ian Stevenson's[1] student and professor of psychiatry and neuropsychology, Jim B. Tucker, and other health professionals from Brazil and Germany. What caught my attention was that the organizer and host of this event was a German person who would repeatedly communicate that the only way to interpret experiences of mediumship is through the teachings of Allan Kardec and that the German scene of spirit-healers would have to (re)turn to Kardecism. He related to hearing voices or perceiving surrounding spirits and introduced techniques to train such a sixth sense. I became aware of the European roots of Spiritism and realized that it is not a sole Brazilian phenomenon but a transnational and -cultural one.

In this chapter, I investigate Spiritism as a translocal practice and discourse of mental healthcare located at the intersection of religion, psychology, and cosmopolitan medicine. It explores central concepts and techniques that may differ from contemporary "Western" psychological and socio-cultural concepts of self, illness, and healing and their adaptation to specific geographical, political, and economic contexts. Divergent interpretations and evaluations illuminate the impact of Spiritist practices and contested positions regarding their benefits for mental health patients in Brazil and beyond. The chapter illustrates the intersection of Kardecism and psychiatry in its historical and culture-specific interrelations and introduces Spiritism as a phenomenon developing partly independently in different parts of the world, focusing on Brazil's extraordinary role in the conservation, transformation, and global (re)distribution of related practices. It will outline the importance Spiritism has gained for the Brazilian healthcare system

DOI: 10.4324/9781032637167-2

throughout the 20th century and how proponents engage and position themselves in disputes on the future of psychiatric hospitals. It implies discussing the challenges and shortcomings of healthcare in Brazil, the anti-psychiatric deinstitutionalization process, and the particularities of Spiritist psychiatry. It will do so as an interdisciplinary literature review, collecting and connecting accounts of anthropologists, sociologists, historians, scholars of religion, psychologists, health professionals, political institutions, and Spiritist experts. The aim is to analyze and interpret culture-specific developments and critically outline controversial debates over space and time. The discussion covers over 200 years of translocal Spiritism, taking its departure in Germany.

Translocal Spiritism

Spiritism and psychiatry are two sides of the same coin: both institutions developed at the dawn of European modernity and the upcoming age of Enlightenment in the late 18th century. They respond to Cartesian perspectives on the human person as an individual and rational being consisting of divergent spheres of the body as the site of emotion and sensuality and the mind hosting rational thought. However, as we will see, the models of a human person differ in spiritual terms, and extraordinary experiences run different risks of being labeled as abnormal or "mad."

In the age of reason and progress, psychiatry as a scientific discipline and therapeutic practice evolved to exclude nonconformity from public discourse and interaction (cf. Foucault 1988a), and psychiatric institutions and asylums served the sake of separating the "abnormal" from the "normal" (Devereux 1980) in terms of rational thought and individual self-responsibility. Accordingly, the rising medical discipline of psychiatry became the tip of the scale defining normal and sanctioning abnormal behavior. "Madness" would not derive anymore from external spiritual agencies (God, Satan, spirits, or demons) but from internal biological or psycho-social dysfunctions. Throughout the subsequent centuries, related therapeutic interventions developed, contested, transformed, and conquered the world in the carry-on baggage of European colonizers (cf. Shorter 1997). Simultaneously, "religion" also experienced rationalization processes, and the Christian model of the human being as a unity of body and soul altered (cf. Porter 1987: 16f). Spiritism and Spiritualism as transcultural phenomena reflected these dynamics. They integrated diverse cultural, philosophical, scientific, religious, and spiritual responses to socio-political challenges of Enlightenment, industrialization, and technological progress (cf. Gutierrez 2015). From a psychological perspective, contemporary discourse on spirits' agencies reflected cultural fears, boundaries, and bigotries, and the trance state of a medium served their communication in terms of "higher" insights (ibid.: 2f). From a historical perspective, Anglo-Saxon Spiritualism and

German-French Spiritism have been vanguards for progressive social reforms at the intersection of religion and politics, e.g., when spirits communicated their critique on gender, class, or race conflicts through human mediums. Related movements can thus be regarded as spiritual companions of Marxism, reflecting contemporary revolutionary ideas on tolerance and equal rights (cf. Barrow 1986; Sharp 2006). Spiritist and Spiritualist movements of the 19th century also contested contemporary psychiatric discourses on internal organic factors by inculpating the responsibility of external factors. Interestingly, these were located in the spiritual sphere rather than in psycho-social or political-economical dynamics, as contemporary social psychiatrists would argue (cf. Shorter 1997).

"Religious-spiritual" and "rational-scientific" approaches to mental health continuously differentiated throughout the 19th century in Europe and would only "de-differentiate" as Complementary and Alternative Medicines (CAM) by the end of the 20th century (Knoblauch 2009; Kirmayer 2014). In his historical overview of Spiritist movements in Europe and Northern America, Sawicki (2016: 9f) refutes Weberian theories predicting the decline of religion and spirituality correlating with modernization and rationalization. He demonstrates that overall, it was members of the economically and politically uprising educated bourgeoisie that would adapt to Spiritist ideas in times of ongoing industrialization and nation-state-building processes. He further argues that Germany was one of its breeding grounds due to pivotal philosophic and scientific impulses (ibid.: 11). Accordingly, German philosophical circles would consider religious, philosophical, and natural scientific models and thoroughly discuss, contest, and finally elaborate contemporary ideas on the nature of the human spirit as an independent, spiritual, and subtle body (ibid.: 13). In particular, German philosopher Jung-Stilling (1740–1817) speculated about human existence after biological death. He integrated aspects of Mesmeric, Cartesian, and Neoplatonist reflections on human nature to develop a theoretical model of the person consisting of a body, a mind, and a soul. The latter would consist of two ingredients: the "spirit" and an "etheric body" that functions as a medium between material and spiritual realities (ibid.: 18). Three axioms frame Spiritist knowledge: (1) Spirits act in the material world, and by certain ritual practices, they can be forced to act in a certain way, (2) spirits can produce material effects and thus affect the human experience, and (3) humans are not necessarily aware of the spiritual influence on their thoughts and actions (ibid.: 19 f). This philosophical construction adapts to Christian ideas of an afterlife where the soul survives death but also approximates animistic cosmologies regarding spirit-human relationships. It further integrates contemporary natural scientific discussions on the physical laws of "cause and effect" and "energy conversion" as well as esoteric concepts of an energetic fluid that permeates the universe and relates the living to the deceased souls (ibid.: 21f).

Theories on the afterlife and human–spirit interactions corresponded to contemporary socio-political values of progress and individuality, promising eternal life by individual progress throughout many lifetimes (as opposed to salvation through Jesus Christ and eternal life with God, cf. Obst 2009). Sawicki relates these ideas to theological reflections on social and mental processes of individualization and agency, which reinterpret human beings as sovereign individuals rather than surrendering to divine grace (Sawicki 2016: 41f). He differentiates between two main movements envisioning communication with the spirits of deceased individuals: Anglo-Saxon Spiritualism and German-French Spiritism. Spiritualism engages in the communication with the spirits of deceased humans; Spiritism, also referred to as Kardecism, further integrates concepts of *karma* and reincarnation, and thus the idea of human souls/spirits progressing from one lived existence to another (ibid.: 19). It seems tempting to interpret the latter as an integration of Eastern religious traditions due to an orientalist enthusiasm of that era, but the concept of soul transmigration does not automatically respond to Hinduism or Buddhism. On the contrary, it differs in many aspects (cf. Obst 2009). For example, German philosophers Jung-Stilling (1740–1817), Lessing (1729–1781), and Goethe (1749–1832) do not perceive reincarnation as a cycle of suffering but as a path toward harmony and happiness and as a possibility to develop personal skills throughout many lifetimes (Sawicki 2016: 48).

German medical doctor Franz Anton Mesmer (1734–1815) was another essential source for Spiritist practice and discourse, particularly regarding healing. According to him, manipulating subtle fluid substances in the patient by laying on hands resolves inner blockades and supports self-healing capacities. Some of his followers reinterpreted these fluids as spiritual influences, and they invented trance-inducing hypnotic practices to learn more about their origin and nature by directly communicating with their alleged sources (ibid.: 134f). Brandt (2014) identifies Mesmerism as an approach to bridge the gaps of an upcoming contemporary differentiation of religious and scientific healing practices by integrating medical and spiritual spheres. Its core element was the concept of animal magnetism as a "fluid" originating from celestial forces, streaming through the human body, and being manipulated by the therapist in terms of "magnetic healing" (Crabtree 2015: 9f). Marquis de Puységur (1751–1825) elaborated related hypnotic techniques and observed that many "magnetized" persons would develop a "sixth sense:" in states of alternate consciousness, they communicated information they were not aware of in "normal states" (ibid.: 10f). Far from discussing it as mediumship, these observations would negotiate psychiatric and spiritual approaches to mental health by acknowledging a religiously informed intrusion paradigm for mental health issues without relating it to religious entities such as God or Satan but as "inner voices" of affecting spirit entities. Since then, Spiritists have explored these approaches, and again, it was German philosopher Jung-Stilling who influenced this enterprise with his argument of the human being as simultaneously living in the material and spiritual world and that "mediums" (so-called "somnam-bulists") would have access to the latter: through magnetization, the soul would become free from its ties to the brain and the nervous system, a state he would call the "perception without bodily senses" (Crabtree 2015: 13). However, due to the positivistic and hegemonical nature of evolving biomedicine in the 19th century, attempts failed to integrate these potentials for innovative healing practices. Instead, spirit communication by self-declared mediums became a more entertainment-oriented practice (ibid.: 14f). With ongoing commercialization, boundaries between Spiritism, Theosophy, and Occultism increasingly dissolved (Sawicki 2016: 243f), and due to the lack of a philosophical and scientific backup, Spiritism and Spiritualism declined in Germany on the eve of World War I. The remaining fire pockets were finally extinguished throughout the German fascist regime and World War II. They would only gradually start to glimmer again with the New Age movement of the 1970s (ibid.: 312f).

In France, the development of Spiritism took a different stance. French scholar Hippolyte Léon Denizard Rivail (1804–1869), with the synonym of Allan Kardec, created a Spiritist doctrine that has ever since been referred to as Kardecism and gained increasing global importance throughout the 20th century (cf. Aubrée & Laplantine 2009). The experiences of Enlightenment, revolution, and reactionism produced cultural-specific perspectives on human and social suffering and progress: individuals would have to fight for their legal rights, salvation, and a society devoid of injustice, poverty, and misery. In this context, Kardec's ideas blended with the socialist visions of Anglo-Saxon Spiritualist Andrew Jackson Davies (1826–1910) insofar as he argued for progress toward a perfect world. However, he also stressed individual responsibility to reach this goal through the moral development of an ideal soul as the result of personal effort and progress throughout many lifetimes (cf. Sharp 2006, 2015): Kardec preached solidarity, charity, fraternity, and moral development. While his doctrine also lost its influence in France on the eve of World War I, in Latin America, and especially in Brazil, its seeds fell on fertile ground throughout the 20th century. According to Sharp (2015: 221f), prospects of progressive development appeared promising to people living in the European colonies with their experiences of structural violence and social stratification. Moreover, to a certain degree, Spiritist concepts of reincarnation and spiritual progress would also corre-spond to local Indigenous and Afro-Brazilian cosmologies (cf. Stubbe 1987; Engler & Brito 2016).

So, what is the core of Kardec's doctrine, and why has it been so central to mental well-being and health? According to his Spirits' Book (Kardec 1996), the human soul disconnects from the biological body upon death and remains in the spiritual realm until reincarnating in a new body for continuous moral development and correcting past-life errors. It does not bear any irony that this religiously informed approach contained contemporary revolutionary and socialist values: all humans are equal in their obligation to progress spiritually. Material privileges and specific social and economic conditions do not derive from any God-given or birthright superiority but serve the need of the incarnate spirit to learn lessons (Sawicki 2016: 287f). Kardec combined persisting post-revolutionary hopes for social reforms and fashionable oriental concepts regarding human spirituality: he fused the wish of an individually, autonomously, and self-responsibly conducted life with postulations regarding social progress toward free will, equality, merit, justice, and tolerance for everybody devoid of class, gender, or race boundaries (ibid.: 223f). Even though Kardec communicated these insights as spiritually transmitted universal laws, his discourse reflected contemporary intellectual influences like, for example, Rousseau (1712–1778), Pestalozzi (1746–1827), and Mesmer (1734–1815). He proclaimed the importance of communication with spirits for education, knowledge, and moral instruction and collected, analyzed, and codified mediumistic messages in his subsequent works. Thus, he redirected Spiritist practice from a light-hearted parlor game toward a scientific-religious search for the truth of the human and spiritual existence in different lifeworlds (ibid.: 232). He defined (spiritual) progress as an increasing moral, selfless, knowledge-oriented, and less materialistic life conduct where self-care would not derive from satisfying desire or vanity but requires care for others: "[t]he concept of advanced spirits aiding those less so echoes that of bodhisattvas and shows to unacknowledged, probably unconscious, blending of eastern ideas into Spiritist thought" (Sawicki 2016: 234).

Kardec aimed at scientifically investigating paranormal experiences and tried to conceive them by exploring, analyzing, and structuring mediumistic communications with spirits (Sawodny 2003: 9). In his Spirit's Book (Kardec 1996), he elaborated 1019 questions and answers from alleged spirits of deceased humans – some of them historical characters – regarding the human–spiritual existence. He developed a cosmology comprising a reinterpretation of the New Testament in the Christian Bible. Accordingly, Jesus Christ was a highly developed spirit (and medium for other spirits) who, after several reincarnations, provided new guidelines for human life and interaction: charity, forgiveness, compassion, humility, generosity, and the avoidance of negative feelings such as pride, envy, animosity, and malice (cf. Sawodny 2003: 13). The concept of reincarnation is crucial: throughout several subsequent incarnations of the immortal spirit/soul within mortal material bodies, the spirit learns how to deal with issues of hostility, guilt and other interpersonal problems which are transported from one lifetime to another until being resolved. Avoiding concepts of "guilt," "remorse," and "punishment," Kardec refers to the physical law of "cause and effect" and the philosophical "law of free will" to characterize human existence as a series of life choices (ibid.: 14f). However, spiritual progress still serves another end: some deceased spirits stay attached to the material world of the living, in particular to those they shared affective ties and/or have had to resolve issues with. This way, they not only block their spiritual progress but also afflict the living. For the sake of their and their human target's benefit, these spirits must be supported in a caring way. Different levels of human moral development would attune to similar spiritual energies, and accordingly, humans would always be surrounded by different spirits that inspire them to behave in certain ways. Similar spirits would attract each other, meaning that discarnate spirits might seek a connection with incarnate spirits on the same energetic level (ibid.: 16f). One way to cut this connection is for afflicted persons to change their behavior, moral habits, and, therefore, energetic level. Another possibility is communicating with the "obsessing" spirit through a medium, a living person who sensory perceives the spirit's presence and transmits messages from the spiritual world (ibid.: 19f). In Brazil, this skill of spirit-human communication has been elaborated throughout the 20th century and is essential to Spiritist mental healthcare.

Spiritism in Brazil

In the second half of the 19th century, various Spiritist practices and discourses reached Latin America and, to a certain degree, mixed with local religions and philosophies (Monroe 2015: 248). The fact that Kardec codified his insights in a series of books reinforced his impact on the further development and global transmission of Spiritism. His doctrine mainly applied to people's quest for a new spiritual practice that connects religious belief with scientific knowledge within challenging and promising new environments:

> To investigate the French origins of Spiritism, therefore, is to place oneself at a fulcrum point in the transnationalisation of Modern Spiritualism as a whole: a moment when a broadly Protestant, highly individualistic, and often radically reformist religious ideology assumed a form more congenial to audiences who shared the American craving for a spiritual practice that seemed to reconcile faith and science, but whose religious assumptions, social visions, and political situations looked very different.
>
> (Monroe 2015: 252)

Kardec attempted to integrate scientific, philosophical, and religious ideas into a system that focuses on the relations between the visible world of humans and the invisible world of spirits as a science dealing with the nature, origin, and destiny of spirits and their relationship with the corporeal world. He systematized his observations following rationalist and scientific conceptions of 19th-century Europe, and they soon crossed the Atlantic to the colonies, where they first gained popularity with European members of the local elites. In Brazil, Kardecism soon became significant in the preexisting diverse Spiritist movements, engendering disputes involving politics, inter-religious relations, and health (Aureliano & Cardoso 2015: 275f).

The First Brazilian Spiritist Congress of 1881 in Rio de Janeiro initiated the foundation of the *Federação Espírita do Brazil* (FEB, "Spiritist Federation of Brazil") in 1884, which has become an umbrella organization for Kardecists in Brazil. Initially, it served the recognition of Spiritism as an official religion, finally being affirmed by the Brazilian government in 1966 also due to their willingness to cope with existing social power structures and the Catholic Church (Aureliano & Cardoso 2015: 278f; cf. Stoll 2003). The case of Francisco Cândido "Chico" Xavier (1910–2002) serves as an example of this political reorientation of Spiritism (cf. Lewgoy 2001): the devoted Catholic became Brazil's most famous Spiritist medium and due to his charitable engagement is nowadays randomly referred to as the reincarnation of enlightened individuals such as Mahatma Gandhi, Jesus Christ, Allan Kardec, or Francis of Assisi. Having almost gained the status of a Brazilian national saint, in 1981, he was nominated for the Nobel Peace Prize. His merit was to communicate alleged messages from the dead and thus provide consolation, hope, and comfort to the surviving mourners. Although never adequately educated and supposedly illiterate, Xavier became famous for his "psychographic" skills, transmitting messages from the spiritual world via automatic writing. Together with his "ghostwriters" (spiritual co-authors), he published several hundred psychographic books and sold over 20 million copies worldwide, donating the revenues to charitable organizations (Aureliano & Cardoso 2015: 278f). Allegedly together with the spirit of the deceased Brazilian journalist, author, and politician Humberto de Campos (1886–1934), Xavier published the book *Brazil, Heart of the World, Homeland of the Gospel* (Xavier 1938), which directly refers to Kardec's (2008) *Gospel According to Spiritism*. Its reinterpretation of biblical accounts and parables draws a picture of Brazil as the spiritually chosen country to preserve, develop, and redistribute the Spiritist legacy globally. Accordingly, all the ethnic, social, religious, political, and economic challenges would finally serve the need for spiritual development and are, therefore, justified as a means to pave the way for Brazil to become a spiritual resource of the world. The conviction of being a spiritual lighthouse and sheet anchor to the rest of the world is widespread even among Brazilians who do not denominate to Spiritism. It is based on the alleged typical Brazilian virtues of love and affection being broadly celebrated in Brazilian popular culture but remaining an ideal in everyday life due to structural violence in the shapes of inequality, violence, and corruption. Even though Brazilian Spiritists engage in over-coming these issues (see Chapter 3), Xavier's discourse still reveals a particular attachment to the political elites of Brazil by trying to justify problematic historical facts – such as the extinction of Indigenous people and the enslavement of Africans – as necessary steps toward a future utopia (cf. Pierini 2020 for the example of *Vale do Amanhecer*).

Chico Xavier successfully promoted Kardecism in Brazil and inspired other authors. Throughout the 20th century, more than 1600 Spiritist books were published in Brazil, thus being the country with the most extensive production of Spiritist literature in the world (Stoll 2003: 50f). The distribution of Spiritist knowledge also adapts to new technologies and the emergence of diversified media resources responds to an increasing request for easy access to spiritual care. In some cases, they even transform from charitable to profitable care services, subverting the original idea of care as self-care (cf. Stoll 2002) and promoting new amalgams with New Age movements that neglect the authority of "traditional" Spiritists (cf. Stoll 2004, 2005). Whereas some Brazilian researchers proclaim Spiritism as a religion of humaneness (Santos 2004), others stress its importance regarding anti-religious and pro-scientific discourses (Terra 2011; Prandi 2013). Giumbelli (1994) addresses the religious-scientific contest within Brazilian Spiritism as an ongoing dispute between divergent agents following different aims, particularly when relating to the increasing engagement with healing and its historic prosecution as an illegal medical practice in the first half of the 20th century (cf. Maggie 2007). Some Spiritists have related to natural scientific discourses like energy transformation, intersubjective connectivity, and even quantum physics to legitimize their spirit-related therapeutic practices. Others propagate the integration of oriental practices like Reiki, Yoga, and meditation, whereas FEB denounces any therapeutic approach and suggests a strict moral and religious reorientation that produces health and well-being in terms of strengthening the spirit and, thus, body and mind (cf. Maggie 1992). The opposing strategies both aim to legitimize Spiritist practice, one appropriating scientific discourse to justify therapeutic practices corresponding to medical standards, the other claiming a space beyond academic medical treatment as religious-spiritual support. Lewgoy (2006a) confirms that the affiliation of Spiritism with ideas of "rationalization" and "scientification" resonates with the upper and more educated classes of Brazil but also states that for many Brazilians, the spheres of "religion" and "science" would not be exclusive but complementary categories, in particular when it comes to resolving everyday life challenges. Accordingly, Spiritism constitutes a unique cultural practice that responds to conditions in the Brazilian healthcare system affecting all Brazilians, negotiating spiritual, biomedical, and psychiatric approaches (Lewgoy 2006b: 152). Moreover, with the New Age movement since the 1970s, Brazilian Spiritist therapeutic approaches also have (re)engaged on a transnational level (Lewgoy 2006a: 174f; see Chapter 5).

The emergence of Spiritism in Brazil coincided with the professionalization and rationalization of medical institutions in demarcation to "traditional" and "faith" healing, persecuted as quack medicine (Luz 2014). Still, Aureliano and Cardoso (2015: 284) argue that this ongoing dispute, at long last, stimulated the production of knowledge on both sides. Again, Chico Xavier and his "ghostwriters" Emmanuel and André Luiz significantly impacted the rapprochement of medical and spirit doctors, elaborating a theoretical and practical frame for Spiritist healing practices. André Luiz is the main character of Xavier's most famous work, *Nosso Lar* ("Our Home," Xavier 1944), which, over half a century later, as a movie (Assis 2010), became a blockbuster in Brazil. The storyboard explores the life and death of medical doctor André Luiz, who developed from a suffering and afflicting spirit to a helping and caring spiritual guide. He became the inhabitant of a colony in the spiritual sphere with a hospital where afflicted and afflicting spirits are treated. This image is essential to *disobsession*, a mediumship practice that intends to heal both the spiritually afflicted humans and the afflicting spirits (see Chapters 3 and 4).

Even though engaging with human–spirit interactions such as practices of mediumship, Kardecists successfully confronted legal accusations of promoting psycho-pathological ideas threatening social hygiene and public health (cf. Giumbelli 1994: 274f), prejudices that were successfully cultivated against Afro-Brazilian practices (Kurz 2013: 43f). Instead of seeking common grounds regarding spiritual care and well-being, FEB delimited from their magical and subversive agencies. This double-strategy of diplomatic negotiation with the political elites and demarcation from Afro-Brazilian practices produced a discourse that distinguishes between "lower" and "real" Spiritism (cf. Giumbelli 2003): even though Afro-Brazilian religions such as *Candomblé* and *Umbanda* would take their steps in the right direction, only Kardecism could provide the correct responses to spiritual and socio-political challenges in Brazil. Throughout the fascist regimes of Getúlio Vargas (1934–1954, with interruptions) and the military dictatorship (1964–1985), Kardecists have increased their ideological influence within various state institutions and claimed for themselves the moral capacity to resolve the malcontents of Brazilian modernity (Giumbelli 1994: 275f). Evidently, these developments reproduced racist and paternalistic structures in Brazilian society, and they did so not only among Kardecists.

Until today, social scientists contest the existence of a "Spiritist continuum" (Camargo 1961) that comprises *Candomblé*, Kardecism, and *Umbanda* as a "real Brazilian religion" fusing African, European, Asian, and Indigenous spiritual practices. It is questionable how far methods of *Candomblé* and *Umbanda* can be equaled to Kardecism due to different socio-cultural, ethnic, formal, and praxeological aspects and, therefore, in how far all these practices can be compiled under the label of "Spiritism" (Aureliano & Cardoso 2015: 279f). Figge (1973: 25) states that mutual saturation exists but that whereas in Kardecism, humans would indoctrinate spirits, in *Umbanda*, spirits would advise humans. Unfortunately, he oversees the rich amount of psychographic Spiritist literature that serves humans' instruction, which is central to the Kardecist practice of evangelization (see Chapter 3). Montero (1985) takes another perspective and interprets *Umbanda* as a popular counterculture to a hegemonic scientific-rationalist discourse, which, on the other hand, Kardecists affiliate with (cf. Hess 1991). However, many *Umbanda* communities would link their Afro-Brazilian roots to Kardecist discourse and practice, developing therapies that complement conventional cosmopolitan medicine with "traditional" phytotherapy and religious-spiritual aspects and support a sense of self-empowerment and agency that addresses both health and social issues (Montero 1985: 253f). In this regard, Brown (1986, 1999) stresses social background, cultural identity, and related class interests in Brazil as factors of religious denomination, whereas Scharf da Silva (2004) and Motta (2005) underline the importance of ritualized bodily performances and aesthetic manipulation that diverge among different approaches independently from their adepts' ethnic and social affiliations. Afro-Brazilian religions and Kardecism would not vary so much in terms of cognitive systems of belief or moral values, but in the way, the human body and senses are addressed and integrated into these practices (Lynch 2005; Hageman et al. 2010; see Chapter 4). Accordingly, Kardecists like to state that they "apply techniques," whereas in *Umbanda*, "they perform rituals" (personal communication by various interlocutors). They ignore the fact that *Umbanda* emerged as a branch of Kardecism after a mediumistic session in the 1920s in Rio de Janeiro, where an alleged mediumistically incorporated spirit postulated the integration of Indigenous, Afro-Brazilian, and European spiritual knowledge (Prandi 2013: 94f).

Surveys of the *Instituto Brasileiro de Geografia e Estatística* (IBGE, "Brazilian Department of Geography and Statistics") reveal demographic and social aspects that elucidate factors of individual affiliations with divergent Spiritist institutions. Based on self-declaration, they investigate the impacts of ethnicity and geographic locality on categories such as social status, education, income, and, to a lesser degree, religious denomination (IBGE 2000, 2011). Synthesizing all these aspects, it appears unreasonable to discuss affiliation with various branches of Spiritism as related to ethnicity/race, gender/sex, or social/economic class (cf. Schmidt 2016a: 47f). On the contrary, I am convinced that the main impetus to engage with Spiritism is a momentary human condition that only partially reflects questions of ethnicity and socialization but manifests a coping strategy and capacity to (re)interpret individual experiences of "otherness." Accordingly, the internal Spiritist differences and conflicts intersect with the diversification of healthcare in Brazil. Hess (1991) observes a gradual integration of religion, spirituality, and medicine among individual practitioners and proclaims the "Brazilian new age in religion, science and medicine" (ibid.: 2) with a plentitude of alternative therapies. He values the capacity to negotiate between institutionalized medical science and folk religious healing as an example of dialogue between non-Western "traditional" and Western "modern" approaches. In a way, he anticipates Bhabha's (1994) theoretical model of a "Third Space" of contest, interaction, and cooperation of healing practices but, unfortunately, does not further investigate social implications and parameters for the emerging diversifying healthcare markets, such as availability, social change, personal networks, and individual decision making of patients (cf. Giumbelli 2008; Schmidt 2017). Instead, he focuses on the professional and institutional level, stating that

> [m]eanwhile, the emergence of transcultural psychiatry in the United States and Europe [...] provided a new way for medical professionals to think about religious healers, and in 1968 the International Symposium on Transcultural Psychiatry was held in Salvador da Bahia, the traditional locus of Afro-Brazilian religions. After this, the medical profession in Brazil increasingly began to concede that the spirit mediumship religions could have therapeutic effects [...].
>
> (Hess 1991: 168f)

Hess describes the interaction between cosmopolitan medical doctors and psychiatrists with Spiritist mediums as ambivalent: the assessment as a psychopathic danger for society would give way to the curiosity on coping strategies and finally to the subversion of long-standing hierarchies that have ignored the well-being of patients (ibid.: 169). Accordingly, a space of gradual integration and cooperation emerged where biomedicals reluctantly opened up to Spiritist practices as complementary "symbolic therapies" (ibid.: 172f). Greenfield takes a similar line of argument and interprets Spiritist healing practices as performative acts where mediums would reenact incidents of previous life experiences that have caused patients' current physical and emotional symptoms. The subsequent indoctrination of the patients and external spiritual agents would help the former reflect on their life conduct and resolve alleged spiritual issues. He emphasizes the psychosocial aspects of Spiritist healing practices where "ritual dramas" symbolize patients' illness experiences and simultaneously transform their interpretations and meanings (Greenfield 1992). In considering a "cultural-biological" model (Greenfield 2008), he assumes increased suggestibility through certain body practices affecting body–mind processes and self-healing capacities. He mentions the existence of typical Spiritist body schemes that support the production of alternative states of consciousness (ASC) but, unfortunately, does not provide detailed information on their operation and functionality. Dilthey (1993: 96f) adds an economic aspect: Spiritist institutions attract patients not so much due to evidence of healing but to the lack of affordable and sustainable alternative resources. However, Brazilian Spiritists also attract foreign patients seeking holistic approaches or at least a spiritual complement to cosmopolitan medicine, especially in cases of chronic illness and adverse therapy outcomes of conventional therapies (cf. Rocha 2017).

Greenfield (1992, 2008) and Dilthey (1993) have mainly explored cases of mediums incorporating spirits of deceased medical doctors, and in particular German ones, such as "Dr. Fritz," who performed surgeries without anesthesia or hygienic precaution. Nowadays, these practices are prohibited but still, mediums of other, mainly German (e.g., Dr. Hans in Ilheus/Bahia, Dr. Hermann in Araraquara/São Paulo, Dr. Frederik in Vitória/Espírito Santo, Dr. Wilhelm in Marília/São Paulo) and Brazilian (Dr. Claudionor in Itabuna/Bahia) deceased medical doctors perform "spiritual surgeries" on the *perispirit* of their patients (see Chapter 5). For several years, Rocha (2017) has accompanied the probably most famous contemporary example, João de Deus ("John of God") in Abadiânia/Goiás, who until recently has attuned to both bodily and spiritual surgeries to treat patients from all over the world. Exploring the social and cultural forces that made this local Brazilian healer a "global guru in the 21st century" (ibid.: 4), Rocha concludes that his healing practices would apply to international New Age concepts, requests, and cultural frames. Questioning the idea of "culture" in this regard, Rocha aptly criticizes Greenfield and his "cultural-biological" model,

> [...] that equates culture with nation, and singles out 'Brazilian culture' as the reason for the efficacy of [...] spiritual surgeries. For him, Brazilians easily enter altered states of consciousness, and once they are 'hypnotized' they are able 'to control pain and alter their flow of blood [...]. In contrast to Western culture, they are assumed to be easily hypnotized because belief in spirits is part of 'Brazilian culture' [...].
>
> (Rocha 2017: 19)

Justifiably, Rocha criticizes this homogenization of national culture and postulates a differentiated perspective that implies dynamic processes of global hybridization and interrelation, especially since so many foreigners adapt to John of God's healing practices (ibid.: 20). She argues that flows of practice and discourse do not only stream from the global North to the global South but multi-directional. As a motivation to turn to Spiritism, Rocha (2017: 8) assumes disillusionment with biomedicine, especially regarding chronic illness experiences and the asymmetric relations between healers and patients. She stresses the empowerment of patients in their quest for the meaning of illness beyond the categories and frames of biomedical technologies. Prandi (2013) agrees when he argues that as an institution, Kardecism in Brazil simultaneously criticizes, substitutes, and complements official health resources by adding spiritual components that address members of all social strata. It substitutes failed public health programs and strategies and provides spaces of agency and self-responsibility at the intersection of charity, care, and education (ibid.: 59f).

Even though not pursuing economic interests, Spiritists acquire their followers through popular mass media and culture industry (ibid.: 75), such as movies, books, journals, television documentaries, and even *telenovelas*, the Brazilian soap operas that attract millions of spectators daily. Kardecism, therefore, plays a significant role in the growing religious-therapeutic marketplace of Brazil (cf. Greenfield 2016). However, apart from economic questions, Brazilians choose healing and spiritual support institutions in a trial-and-error strategy and affiliate with those that best serve their needs and where they feel well-treated (Rabelo 2005). This way, throughout the 20th century, Kardecism has become a serious player within the Brazilian (mental) healthcare system and beyond. Rocha (2017) stresses the increasingly transnational character of Spiritism not only regarding the "medical tourism" of foreigners traveling to Brazil but translocal transportation by Brazilian migrants. Lewgoy (2008) states that this is particularly true for the branch of Kardecism that, through the guidance and global mission of FEB, has followers in over thirty countries, particularly in Europe. On the one hand, Kardecist institutions support Brazilian migrants adapting to new contexts, but on the other hand, they also address increasing numbers of non-Brazilian adepts and face processes of "de-Brazilianization" (see Chapter 5).

Spiritism and Mental Healthcare

The anthropological discussion and psychological interpretation of Brazilian Spiritist practices as mental health resources illuminate a recent discourse and indicate a paradigmatic shift regarding the intersection of spiritual well-being and health throughout the second half of the 20th century (cf. Silva de Almeida et al. 2007; Isaia 2010). Before, in particular, Afro-Brazilian practices were labeled psycho-pathologically as "collective madness" and "irrational behavior" (Guedes 1974: 86f, 185), and throughout the early 20th century, this prejudice extended to Kardecism (cf. Ribeiro & de Campos 1931). As a counter-reaction to increasing neglect by scientific institutions and simultaneously applying to contemporary scientific discourse on energy transmission, Spiritists developed and elaborated nosologies of mental, emotional, and spiritual distress as results of malevolent spiritual and energetic influences (Guedes 1974: 92f). Accordingly, even though Afro-Brazilian traditions held a more vital position in the Brazilian society, it was thus mainly 20th-century Kardecism that in both cooperation and contest with cosmopolitan psychiatry produced relevant alternative and complementary theories on mental health disorders (Moreira-Almeida & Lotufo Neto 2005: 572).

Kardec was interested in the etiology of the spirit world and its relationship to the world of the living, but in his *Journal of Psychological Studies* (1858–1869), he also studied cases of behavioral disorders, suicide attempts, and shifts of sensory perception. He did not reject biological, psychological, or social explanatory models of mental disorder but added spiritual aspects in terms of negative influences of discarnate spirits (*obsession*) to the list of possible causes. He assumed organic reasons as the primary etiology of mental disorders that would only attract obsessing spirits in a second step. Accordingly, and in contrast to subsequent approaches, Kardec did not recommend mediumship training as a therapeutic practice. He was convinced that physical or mental imbalances of a patient/medium would attract more malevolent than benevolent spirits (ibid.: 570f). Even though he added the spiritual sphere to his model of a human person, Kardec responded to the Cartesian mind/body model with the slight difference that beyond being superior to the material body, the spirit/mind would be independent of it. However, he assumed a mutual influence of bodily and mental processes and stated that immoral/abnormal behavior would cause obsession by malevolent spirits. Accordingly, Kardec discussed the explanatory model of "spiritual obsession" as a symptom of, rather than a cause for, mental disorders. Therapeutic approaches henceforth would then have to integrate attempts to transform the patient's behavior toward moral growth, supported by practices of laying on hands (*passe*), study, prayers, and the establishment of rapport with obsessing spirits in mediumistic sessions (ibid.: 575f).

Bezerra de Menezes (1920) integrated this philosophy with early Brazilian mental healthcare discourse, wondering if there might be alternative explanations to "human madness" than organic brain defects. Having studied philosophical literature on human existence and Kardec's works, he concluded that discarnate spirits would act upon the living via "fluidal action." According to his argument, humans consist of a spirit (soul) and a body connected by the human brain (mind). The spirit would disconnect from the biological body upon death but might not cease to affect other bodies in terms of obsession or fluidly interrupting and influencing the spirit-brain-communication of afflicted persons (ibid.: 65f). Transgressing Kardec's theoretical approaches, Bezerra de Menezes thus postulated that "madness" could be *either* due to organic dysfunction causing obsession *or* obsession causing organic dysfunction (ibid.: 120f). Differential diagnosis thus must be obtained by hypnotizing patients, evoking obsessors, and consulting protective spirits in mediumistic sessions (Moreira-Almeida & Lotufo Neto 2005: 581). Not being a psychiatric practitioner, Bezerra de Menezes still suggested that since there were twofold causes of insanity, treatment modalities should also be differentiated (ibid.: 582). The first Brazilian psychiatrist to turn this theory into practice was Inácio Ferreira de Oliveira (1904–1988), director of the *Sanatório Espírita de Uberaba* ("Spiritist Sanatorium of Uberaba" in Minas Gerais) from 1934 to 1988. He implemented a combined treatment, including mediumship training and the participation of patients in mediumistic sessions (cf. Jabert 2011). Following this new model of orientation in Brazilian psychiatry, between 1930 and 1970, about 50 Kardecist psychiatric hospitals evolved in Brazil (Moreira-Almeida & Lotufo Neto 2005: 572). With some modifications, Spiritist mental healthcare institutions in Brazil have implemented this approach until today, and many honor Bezerra de Menezes as a spiritual mentor.

The Brazilian medium and long-time figurehead of the Brazilian Spiritist Federation (FEB), Divaldo Pereira Franco (*1927), has developed a divergent approach, linking Kardecist theories to transpersonal and Jungian psychology. He does not neglect spirit obsession as a cause of mental health disorders but stresses the impact of spirits' experiences in current and past lives on patients' thoughts, acts, and behavior through the unconscious. Ethical behavior, introspection, and moral reflection would generate health capacities of the spirit that also affect the body (cf. Moreira-Almeida & Lotufo Neto 2005: 585). Franco published more than 150 psychographic books, some translated into up to 15 languages, promoting and representing a contemporary Kardecist mainstream in and outside Brazil (ibid.: 584). However, even though he refers to cases of obsession (Franco 2010) and other spiritual aspects of emotional disturbances (Franco 2009), he fails to define explanatory and therapy models. Instead, he preaches "moral behavior" and spiritual progress as guidelines to deal with neurosis (ibid.: 17f), psychosis (ibid.: 31f), schizophrenia (ibid.: 77f), or depression (ibid.: 105f).

In addition to social, biological, or psychological factors of mental health affliction, he stresses three interrelated aspects: (1) organic causes that respond to medical treatment, (2) spiritual aspects are always involved, and their solution supports medical treatment, and (3) the concept of reincarnation is the key to understand these aspects (ibid.: 12f). The spirit of a patient would reincarnate to develop morally and to compensate past mistakes, but obsessive menace (ibid.: 17f) and dynamics of self-punishment for evil deeds in past lives (ibid.: 31f) would disturb this process. Obsessors seek revenge and transfer their trauma to whom they hold responsible for their misery, and the combination with feelings of guilt affects the energetic body (*perispirit*) of the patient and, therefore, body and mind (ibid.: 47f); in other words: karmic issues produce suffering (ibid.: 90). As a resource for health and well-being, Franco suggests mental hygiene through the lecture of Kardec's (2008) "Gospel According to Spiritism" and the practice of "Christian discipline," such as moral reformation, education, and training "love in the name of Jesus" (Franco 2009: 20f).

In conjunction with Kardec, Bezerra de Menezes, and Xavier, Franco develops a tripartite model of the human person, which consists of a material body, an immaterial spiritual body, and a subtle energetic body (*perispirit*) that connects these spheres. Even though Franco does not define it as a logical consequence, the "mind" is not an independent sphere like in the Cartesian model but a conglomerate of (materially, spiritually, and energetically) embodied experiences and memories of all three bodies. External influences such as religious belief, socialization, political conditions, cultural frames, and biological heritage influence individual psychological and emotional problems, but the disposition is rooted in the reincarnated spirit and imprints itself on the material body via the *perispirit* (ibid.: 112f).

An increasing number of Brazilian medical professionals are Spiritists and organized in the *Associaçao Medico-Espírita* (AME; "Spiritist Medical Association"), integrating these concepts into their scientific research and the daily practice of (mental) healthcare (Moreira-Almeida & Letufo Neto 2005: 572; cf. Teixera Soares 2009). In 1968, AME formed in São Paulo and, by 1991, organized the first Spiritist Medical Congress, since then biannually performed in different Brazilian cities. The 2019 convention in Teresina/Piauí attracted approximately 4000 national and international health professionals and performed as a scientific conference with lectures, workshops, and book tables on the topic of "The Evolution of Spirituality in the Context of Health: Enlarging Ideas and Defeating Paradigms." Members of AME aim to produce medical knowledge through the observation, analysis, and discussion of Spiritist healing practices in reference to cosmopolitan medicine and psychiatry. AME, therefore, attracts an increasing number of academically trained health professionals in their attempt to reconcile scientific and spiritual aspects of therapy (cf. Aureliano & Cardoso 2015: 285). By 1995, nine regional groups of AME already have formed in Brazil, and their umbrella organization "AME-Brasil" has evolved toward an international institution to promote the study of Spiritism as a global health resource (cf. Prandi 2013). By 1999, AME members had established the transnational branch AME-International, promoting worldwide conferences, workshops, social media performances, and extensive media production to distribute Spiritist knowledge as a base for (self-)care and healing (see Chapter 5). AME authors refer to the publications of Kardec, Bezerra de Menezes, Xavier, and Franco to postulate a synthesis of religious and scientific paradigms in a "new era of medicine" (cf. Associação Medico-Espírita 2009). Several dedicate to the psychiatric diagnosis of depression as a result of guilt feelings and past-life errors (cf. Claro 2008), stressing the impact of Kardecist practices as resources in terms of "self-healing" (cf. de Olivieira et al. 2001: 56f). Spiritist psychiatrist Munari (2008) investigates the correlation of psychiatric diagnosis, bodily symptoms, and the function of the *perispirit*. He assumes an impact of obscure physiological materiality, which so far has been ignored within the discipline of psychiatry. He designates it a semi-material substance that he calls "vital fluid" or "ectoplasm" and proposes its importance for the therapy process since it would correspond to the semi-material quality of the *perispirit* (ibid.: 17). Munari observes a correlation of spiritual influences and past-life experiences with the actual overproduction of ectoplasm in psychiatric patients, especially in cases of depression and psychosomatic disturbances (ibid.: 52f, 91f). Mental healthcare, therefore, would also have to address bodily/sensorily aspects of well-being to complement the spiritual-cognitive approaches of mental hygiene, charity, and the practice of love (ibid.: 115f).

Mental Healthcare in Brazil

In Brazil, the so-called "psy-sciences" emerged differently from European dynamics of segregating religious and scientific spheres. Initially, psychology marked a somewhat experimental and interdisciplinary project at the intersection of philosophy, medicine, and theology and only gained the status of an independent scientific discipline in 1932 (Alberti 2003: 14f). Jesuit and Aquinian influences resulted in the integration of the human soul as a central concept contesting Cartesian body–mind models (ibid.: 17f). As a consequence, an oscillation between religiously informed therapy models and the medicalization of psycho-social issues have characterized Brazilian mental healthcare practices throughout the 20th and beginning 21st centuries (ibid.: 22). The emergence of positivism as a republican discourse on order and progress as guidelines for a distinct Brazilian modernity promoted practices of social hygiene and control (ibid.: 22) but still displayed Christian values (ibid.: 25) and, therefore, linked the human constitution to questions of morality (ibid.: 26f). However, the diverse schools of Brazilian psychology would randomly refer to concepts like "conscience," "soul," or "spirit" referring to an external agency apart from body–mind without having to explicitly engage with transcendent institutions such as "God" (ibid.: 39). Different approaches developed to produce a moral body: while some psychotherapists suggested practices of introspection to acquire "inner balance" and "mental hygiene," others would postulate external moralizing interventions (ibid.: 45f). Alberti thus observes a bifurcation between spiritual and materialistic approaches, the latter tending to discriminate and medicalize abnormal behavior (ibid.: 100). They anchor in divergent frames of social class, geographic space, and patterns of religious-cultural socialization and also mirror a contest on the monism vs. dualism of body/mind and soul (ibid.: 104).

Stubbe (1987: 13) adds that from a historical perspective, the concept of the soul and the self in Brazilian psychology does not solely derive from Jesuit thought but integrates Indigenous, Afro-Brazilian, and Christian concepts (ibid.: 16). He describes Brazilian psychology as two intersecting but independently existing currents with Spiritism at the nodal point of mediation: one current represents endogenous religious-ritualistic "ethno-psychologies" of Indigenous Brazilians, Afro-Brazilians, and early Portuguese immigrants, whereas the other displays exogenous modernity in terms of an imported, institutionalized Western academic psychology (ibid.: 19f). Already about 40 years ago, Stubbe (1987: 176) declared the Brazilian mental healthcare system insufficient due to its incapability to provide resources in remote areas and among lower social classes. As a result, religious-spiritual therapies have always substituted insufficient official healthcare approaches providing spaces of solidary care, particularly for the socially disadvantaged (ibid.: 176f). Many official mental health institutions denied related ethno-psychological approaches, and instead of treating and supporting patients for their benefits, until at least the 1980s, Brazilian psychiatry segregated and stigmatized patients as *incapaz* ("unfit") for the rest of their lives (Gattaz & Stubbe 1981: 199f). This inhumane treatment climaxed throughout the political-military regime of Brazil (1964–1985), but over 30 years later, Amarante (2018: 7) still complains that the biggest problem in Brazilian mental healthcare is social exclusion and, therefore, justifies the contemporary Brazilian psychiatry reform that, in line with the 1990 Declaration of Caracas,[2] aims at restructuring psychiatric assistance in line with human rights (cf. Conselho Federal de Psicologia et al. 2018). However, Amarante (2018: 8) doubts that the political strategy of closing psychiatric hospitals and replacing them with so-called *Centros de Atenção Psico-Social* (CAPS, "Psycho-Social Attention Centers") will have the envisioned effect of social inclusion of patients within their communities as long proper basic resources of care remain undistributed (cf. Botega 2002, Paixão Santos & de Oliveira Nunes 2011; Pinto 2015; School 2015). Biehl (2018) also questions the somewhat unilateral view on psychiatric hospitals that frames this discourse. He states that there have been precarious asylums and "zones of abandonment" (ibid. 2005) primarily when affiliated with the official healthcare sector, but also stresses the existence of "good examples" of hospitalized mental healthcare in Brazil, mainly being administered by philanthropic organizations (ibid.: 251). He doubts that redirecting patients and, therefore, the responsibility to families and local communities would resolve the problem. Quite the opposite, particularly in rural areas and lower economic classes, many relatives and community members appreciate facilities to exclude these individuals instead of having to integrate with them on an everyday basis (ibid.: 252f). Nunes and Marques (2018: 11f), in this regard, stress the importance of social relations for patients within a space where they can participate and unfurl; specific patient associations[3] and charitable projects would often better respond to patients' needs and experiences than their local communities (ibid.: 13). Besides structural resources, prejudice and social acceptance of psychiatric diagnosis have been challenges for care and social inclusion (cf. Peluso & Blay 2009). Velpry (2018) suggests art therapy/ production as a means for patients to explore themselves and interact with others, an approach already having been promoted earlier by pioneering psychiatrist Nise Magalhães da Silveira (1905–1999). She initiated projects where marginalized psychiatric patients could express their experiences and publicly exhibit the results (Cerqueira & Felgueiras 2018: 927). In 1956, she would, therefore, establish the *Casa das Palmeiras* ("House of Palm-Trees") in Rio de Janeiro as a deinstitutionalization project for psychiatric patients to reintegrate into society in an open space for in- and outpatients to bridge gaps between the spheres of the mental hospital and society, and at the same time avoid internalization (ibid.: 940). It took another 40 years for the Brazilian government to follow this example and inaugurate the country's first CAPS in São Paulo in 1987 and another 15 years to govern psychiatric reforms (ibid.:

944). Like Amarante, Goulart and Durães (2010: 112) also critically view the psychiatric deinstitutionalization process. The example of the Raul Soares Institute (IRS), a psychiatric hospital in Belo Horizonte/Minas Gerais, illustrates contradictory Brazilian mental healthcare policies and the need for profound and sustained socio-cultural changes to enable a sufficient and adequate future mental healthcare distribution. Their historical overview begins with the common early 20th-century practice of interning patients in concentration camps such as the *Colônia de Barbacena* ("Colony of Barbacena," Minas Gerais). It continues in the 1920s, when subsequent administrations of psychiatric hospitals would, apart from medicalization, oscillate between the implementation of psycho-social assistance and social hygiene by exclusion. The latter being again reinforced after Vargas' fascist revolution in the 1930s, it would take another fifty years until the human degradation in psychiatric institutions again became a focus of popular interest and subsequent postulations of reformation. Since the 1980s, integrative therapeutic communities and ambulances have been established where patients, family members, volunteers, and teams of interdisciplinary therapists work and sometimes even live together (ibid.: 113). This account of Brazilian psychiatric institutions impressively elucidates the issues, challenges, and problems of the Brazilian psychiatry reform at the intersection of medical, social, and political dynamics and forces throughout history.

It also indicates why the Brazilian anti-psychiatry movement has been condemned to failure. Related policies promoted the immediate shutdown of all psychiatric inpatient facilities to counteract strategies to abuse psychiatric institutions for social control. At the same time, they facilitated a market-related boom of private psychiatric clinics. One way or the other, many public psychiatric hospitals closed because they have not adequately and persistently met the challenges of transforming mental healthcare from a segregated toward an integrative therapy model (Goulart & Durães 2010: 118). In his extensive study of a psychiatric hospital in Rio de Janeiro, Brody (1973) already has outlined related socio-cultural markers such as skin color, social status, religion, education, economic status, gender, and age as prominent factors for psychiatric hospitalization in Brazil. With the decline of the military regime, subsequent democratic governments established the *Sistema Única de Saúde* (SUS, "Unitary Health System") in cooperation with non-governmental social movements to overcome such inequalities in (mental) healthcare by the provision of free medical treatment and primary care to everybody. However, Giovanella and Porto (2004) criticize the lack of quality and social control, unequal geographical and social access, fragmentation of institutions and agencies, and decreasing social and political governance scope. They address shortcomings and inconsistencies of SUS, such as failed socio-economic issues – including pressures by the International Monetary Fund (IMF) – explosively population growth in industrialized and urbanized regions, increasing social inequality and asymmetric relations, and chaotic infrastructures. Above all, systemic corruption would impede the vision of an integral bio-psycho-social healthcare system and social participation (ibid.: 36f). Bernardo and Garbin (2011: 103) add further challenges for integrative mental healthcare, e.g., the transformation of workers' healthcare from a culture of stigmatization as a burden of society toward a solidary system valuing persons beyond their capacity to contribute to the labor market (ibid.: 104). Overall, instead of investing in the population's social education and patients' empowerment, new state-controlled institutions emerged: with federal law in 2001, the establishment of CAPS served the political ideology of a progressive extinction of psychiatric hospitals and the autonomy and social inclusion of the mentally afflicted but efforts in prevention, health promotion, and assistance of mental health patients have remained far from being sufficient (ibid.: 105). In many parts of the country, CAPS cannot correspond to the requests for psycho-social assistance due to a lack of cooperation with other healthcare institutions (ibid.: 105f).

The WHO-Aims Report on mental health services in Brazil (WHO 2007) provides details regarding the distribution and reform of mental healthcare in correlation to demographic dynamics and social aspects (ibid.: 6). CAPS and the related Return-Home-Program were designed as innovative services and interventions to abolish custodial care and psychiatric hospitalization in favor of free access to psychotropic drugs and a diversity of outpatient services, day clinics, therapeutic workshops, and community care facilities (ibid: 8). Ever since, the number of inpatient facilities has decreased, and acute conditions are often temporarily treated in general hospitals or under the surveillance of CAPS in cooperation with private psychiatric clinics. However, with 5259 psychiatrists, 12377 psychologists, 11958 social workers, 3119 psychiatric nurses, and 2661 occupational therapists for 188,078,227 psychiatric inpatients in 2007,

> [...] services are unequally distributed across regions of the country, and the growth of elderly population [...] is creating an increased gap in mental health-care. This gap may get even wider if funding does not increase and mental health services are not expanded in the country.
>
> (WHO 2007: 8)

Another major problem is the lack of transparency and communication between the various involved institutions: official documents, programs, annual trends, and plans for future actions, especially regarding child and adolescent mental health, do not exist or have disappeared (ibid.: 8), simultaneously with official funds to improve the healthcare system that absconded in the mills of corruption and bureaucracy (cf. Lewis 2006). In 2005, SUS transposed approximately 15 billion US$, equivalent to 82.7 US$ per capita per year. Of this amount, only 358 million US$ (1.95 US$ per capita and 2.4% of the overall resources) were invested in mental healthcare services. Moreover, a significant reduction from 95.5% to 49.3% of the mental healthcare funds for psychiatric hospitals has not been covered by increases from 0.8% to 15% for community services and from 0.1% to 15.5% for psychotropic medicines since the mid-1990s (WHO 2007: 8f). Furthermore, the lack of psychiatric education in the curricula of general medicine and nursing constitutes a shortage of psychiatric nurses and psychiatrists who moreover are unequally distributed across the country, explicitly leaving less populated and poorer areas without supply (ibid.: 10).

Mateus et al. (2008) provide slightly higher numbers regarding the psychiatric coverage in Brazil but also complain that in a direct comparison of the Southeastern and Northeastern regions of Brazil, a difference of five to one psychiatrist(s) per 100,000 inhabitants occurs (ibid.: 1). On a national scale, around 27 psychiatric beds per 119 patients are available, and an average stay at a psychiatric hospital lasts 65 days, whereas SUS only funds one month. The nationwide 848 CAPS arithmetically have to each cover 200,000 inhabitants but likewise are unequally distributed (ibid.: 1f). In conclusion, the investigators of WHO claim the need for academically trained health managers with knowledge of epidemiology, anthropology, biostatistics, health policy, economics, and planning as an essential investment to achieve coverage, efficiency, and resource utilization (WHO 2007: 10f). In conclusion, the overall judgment of the WHO investigators displays discontent. Besides the economic aspects and the inconsistencies of mental healthcare distribution, another issue to be resolved concerns the surveillance of human rights and the promotion of social solidarity (ibid.: 9). Accordingly, WHO officials urge more self-help programs, patient-family associations, social participation, education, prevention, and health promotion, as well as improvement of monitoring transparency (ibid.: 11f) and long-term studies on the effectiveness of these programs (ibid.: 41).

However, from a medical anthropologist's perspective, the fact that this report does not even mention socio-cultural implications, religious resources, and existing structures of healing cooperation (see Chapter 3) constitutes an obstacle to the profound assessment of the mental healthcare system of Brazil. Unfortunately, the Brazilian Ministry of Health does not provide any enlightening information either: a treatise on the conventional mental healthcare system (Ministério da Saúde 2004) does not present or analyze reliable data but reduces to vaguely promising community-based assistance to substitute hospital-centered therapies (ibid.: 9). It promotes the idea of a network to integrate public and private health-related and social institutions and programs for the sake of warranting daily care, therapy organization, and social inclusion in education, work, sports, culture, leisure, and other activities (ibid.: 11f) but does not present any strategy or concrete initiative on how to realize these aims; it is thus little surprise that a few years later, a review of the progress and problems regarding the psychiatry reform throughout the first government (2003–2006) of President Luiz Inácio "Lula" da Silva admits that many issues have remained unresolved (Ministério da Saúde 2007). It postulates better coordination and surveillance on federal, state, and regional levels, more social participation, and the solution of coverage problems: still, of nationwide 1011 CAPS in 2006, 166 are located in the state of São Paulo (Southeast), 89 in the state of Bahia (Northeast) and only one in the state of Roraima (North) (ibid.: 10f). Regarding the coverage of CAPS per 100,000 inhabitants (nationwide about 0.4), it even corresponds to different population densities, but infrastructure and distance remain obstacles to many patients (ibid.: 14). In 2008, the Brazilian Ministry of Health published another paper concerning the integration of CAM with SUS "for political, technical, economic, social, and cultural reasons" (Ministry of Health 2008: 5). The exact reasons remain unexplained and the promoted therapy models do not include any Brazilian Indigenous, religious, and/or spiritual resources. Instead, they cover, among others, traditional Chinese medicine, acupuncture, homeopathy, phytotherapy, and anthroposophical medicine (ibid.: 3), intending to provide humanized care models based on the integrality of patients (ibid.: 5). It is doubtful whether patients with limited access to health facilities will benefit from this reform; instead, it applies to patients in urban regions with specific resources regarding mobility and flexibility. Moreover, it adapts to recent readjustments of healthcare in Europe and North America without considering specific Brazilian contexts and resources (except for phytotherapy).

Over 40 years ago, Luz (1979: 14f) criticized the official Brazilian health institutions for rejecting therapeutic approaches not being covered by scientific institutions and political interests. According to her, political control and uniformity are characteristic of the Brazilian healthcare system and would not so much orientate toward a better health supply for the population but toward governance and social guidance (ibid.: 18f, 2014). This attitude has met resistance, especially among the poor segments of Brazilian society. Kraatz (2001), for example, performed field research with women in Brazilian *favelas* ("shanty-towns") to explore the distribution and acceptance of official healthcare practices. She observes a contradiction between the constitutional right of free healthcare and the resources provided for the lower classes in Brazil (ibid.: 174), generating denial, doubt, and sometimes even fear of modern medicine (ibid.: 177). She also indicates that religious resources play a significant role in establishing local healthcare facilities (ibid.: 178). Likewise, Caldwell (2017) addresses the structural and institutional inadequacies and failures of healthcare in Brazil, particularly for poor Afro-Brazilian women. Even though she acknowledges progress in health equity since the 1980s due to activists, social initiatives, and scientific work, she criticizes that it is still the poor, the female, and people of color in Brazil who suffer most from structural violence and inequalities in healthcare provision. She focuses on the official Brazilian public health system SUS and explores its strengths and shortcomings concerning gender and racial equity once SUS as a political project has been designed to produce equal treatment for all citizens, regardless of ethnic, social, or gender background. Caldwell criticizes its poor implementation partially due to administrative indifference and corruption (ibid.: 177f). It is the strength of her argument to outline the social, political, and economic abysses within the Brazilian healthcare system, but in my opinion, these issues cannot be reduced to questions of ethnicity and gender: many people in Brazil suffer from insufficient therapy options and if there is any need at all to categorize them, the concept of race should be substituted by class or locality because, as I have elaborated, access to medical treatment does not so much depend on skin color but to infrastructure and economic resources. I do not deny discriminatory practices and discourse in contemporary Brazilian (health) politics, but by exclusively focusing on race and gender, Caldwell does not deliver a representative study of the Brazilian healthcare system. With all her effort to ask the right questions, a more holistic investigation of Brazilian (mental) healthcare is needed.

Leibing (2007) analyzes the Brazilian healthcare system as based on a division between a private high-tech and a public sector, the latter with immense regional variation providing only primary care with long waiting lists and a shortage of material resources and health professionals. According to her, these issues transgress ethnic and cultural distinctions and instead reveal an opposition between urban centers and rural peripheries (ibid.: 59). As a cultural feature, she observes an intense preoccupation with health among the Brazilian population irrespective of their social, cultural, and economic background: in the state of Rio de Janeiro for example, one pharmacy serves 2648 inhabitants (WHO recommends 8000), and Brazil is one of the world's top consumer of pharmaceuticals with two-thirds of them being available without a prescription, including psychotropic remedies (ibid.).

Another peculiarity is the immanent impact of body politics, especially regarding the discursive construction of a "beautiful national body" (ibid.: 62f; cf. Cantalice 2011).[4] Kriesel (2001) stresses the quotidian importance of sensory and bodily experience with an almost religious connotation: skillfulness, beauty, and pleasure have become national symbols for ideal performance of human interaction and are showcased in the carnival, soccer, and beach life where otherwise prominent social differences fade (ibid.: 48f). He argues that the body in Brazil, more than in other cultures, is the locus of social interaction and a symbol of national and individual identity; life's reality would be mainly experienced and communicated through bodily practices and less by cognitive and discursive engagement (ibid.: 62f).[5] Therein, Rödiger (2003) observes "the body" in Brazil as a symbolic matrix of social interaction, experience, emotion, and religious practice. She interprets the presence and performance of an "aesthetic body" in its visual aspects as social capital and a medium to overcome social marginalization, affliction, and passivity. On the other hand, the suffering body also communicates these experiences as illness (Scheper-Hughes 1994). From this perspective, the spiritual interpretation of corporeal experience as an explanatory model for illness (cf. Kleinman 1988a,b) and idioms of distress (cf. Nichter 1981, 2010) within Brazilian mental healthcare deserves consideration. For example, Rabelo and Souza (2003: 333) discuss the concept of *nervos*[6] as a bodily symptom related to difficult life circumstances. Suffering from *nervos* cannot be reduced to a "somatization" of psycho-social affliction but is a cultural idiom of embodying and communicating experiences of powerlessness and impotence, especially among members of the poor and physically exploited hard-working populations (ibid.: 358). In this line of thought, social weakness and poor self-determination are translated into bodily weakness and a lack of self-control. Here, religious practices provide coping strategies, e.g., the transformation of perceived meanings of these experiences. Araújo (1991: 159f) investigates how symptoms like anxiety, insomnia, palpitations, feelings of heat, fatigue, excitability, weakness, and loss of vitality relate to social experiences and do not respond to pharmaceutic treatment. According to local body images and cosmologies, the illness of *nervos* has produced a weak body into which spirits may enter and weaken it more. In *Candomblé*, healers would then work with a principle of power (*axé*) and provide power transmissions to help the body to "close" (ibid.: 162, cf. Rabelo 1993).

The concept of power transmission is comparable to Kardecism, where the practice of *passe* provides positive fluids/energies to the patient. It differs so far that causes of affliction are not externalized as psycho-social issues but internalized in spiritual terms. Even though in both cases, external spiritual agencies have an impact on the patient, in Kardecism, it is the patient's responsibility to spiritually develop and have the spirit indoctrinated and expulsed, whereas in *Candomblé*, a pacification by integration of the spirit is acquired. The point is that Afro-Brazilian religions support individual empowerment by relating to psycho-social and political problems through bodily communication (cf. Kurz 2013; Seligman 2014) and that treating symptoms without addressing their causes is pointless (Araújo 1991: 165). Leibing (1995: 4) criticizes that this correlation of bodily symptoms with psycho-social or spiritual issues has been ignored in Brazilian psychiatry (as a European-generated rational discipline, ibid.: 30). On the contrary, psychiatrists would pathologize bodily (and spiritual) discourse as irrational and invest their effort into convincing patients of cognitive-psychological causes and effects. As a result, bodily symptoms are exclusively treated pharmaceutically, and therapy means adapting to and coping with problems instead of resolving them (ibid.: 44f). Even though Leibing does observe opposition to mere medical treatment by some politically engaged psychiatrists within the investigated psychiatric hospital in Rio de Janeiro, she is critical that patients remain perceived as passive victims of the system without any support of agency or empowerment initiation (ibid: 46f). It is a persisting chronic symptom of psychiatry itself that instead of acknowledging patients as active members of society, their marginal status intensifies, and healthcare institutions manage affliction instead of healing it (ibid.: 55).

Spiritist Psychiatry in Brazil

According to Hess (1991), Spiritist mental healthcare bridges the gap between allegedly opposing religious and psychiatric spheres. On the one hand, efforts aim at overcoming the externalization of causes and stress the patients' responsibility for recovery. In that line, Spiritists argue for a complement to medicalization by the patients' empowerment, agency, and social inclusion. I want to add that Spiritist psychiatry substitutes the lack of resources in the official mental healthcare sector and remains the only resource of inpatient psychiatric treatment resisting the anti-psychiatric deinstitutionalization policy in Brazil. Already half a century ago, Brody (1973: 11) stated that large numbers of mentally afflicted persons would consult Spiritist centers seeking social support in dealing with emotional or bodily issues, anxieties, addictions, or other dysfunctions, receiving either spiritual treatment or the advice to seek medical treatment with spiritual support (ibid.: 414f). He investigated a psychiatric hospital in Rio de Janeiro administrated by a Spiritist association where some patients were treated for free upon mediumistically communicated spirits' instructions. The medical staff would hardly engage with Spiritism, but patients were allowed to frequent a nearby Spiritist center for spiritual support. Brody observes extraordinary progress in those patients who have done so and criticizes the medical staff for ignoring this phenomenon or, if acknowledging it at all, reducing it to the "calming effects" of religious engagement (ibid.: 429f). About 20 years later, Spinu and Thorau (1994) investigated the diagnostic-therapeutic practice of *captação* in a private psychiatric clinic in São Paulo as a transmission of patients' symptoms by Spiritist mediums in cooperation with academically trained psychologists and psychiatrists. Mediums would communicate the spiritual causes of an affliction, and treatments of diagnosed psychosomatic and psycho-social distress have been quite successful. It connects concepts of spirits with the unconscious and spiritual issues with "conflicts of unconscious personalities" to integrate transpersonal psychology with a holistic-dynamical energy model in Spiritism. Afro-Brazilian cosmic and social interrelation concepts are reinterpreted, and states of trance or possession are described as altered states of consciousness (ibid.: 21f). With reference to Carl Gustav Jung (1875–1961), experiences and their communication are dealt with as symbolic forms without neglecting or supporting divergent interpretations but to integrate them into therapy so that patients gain insight into the causes and effects of their affliction and learn how to cope with them (ibid.: 85f, 269f). This approach would help patients to communicate, elaborate, and transform their experience (cf. Redko 2003).

Wiencke (2006) further explores this phenomenon with a focus on Spiritism as a holistic system where social, physical, mental, and spiritual aspects correlate (ibid.: 70): the support of a solidary group would help to cope with an illness and to develop strategies to transform its experience and meaning in terms of a spiritual cosmology, self-image, and habitus. He infers that Spiritist practices are not about healing but dealing with an affliction (ibid.: 71) and its compensation within a supportive social network (ibid.: 78). Making sense of and giving meaning to an illness experience would take its horror (ibid.: 96) and the prospect of being able to develop spiritually and at the same time supporting others in similar processes affect self-perception and interaction with others (ibid.: 116f). Being an anthropologist and psychologist, Wiencke develops what I call a "cognitive-performative" approach where Spiritist practices serve as a form of group therapy (ibid. 2006: 150, 2009) to resolve concealed conflicts within Brazilian social structures and/or local communities (ibid.: 165). He implements Turner's (1982: 61f) perspective on individual affliction corresponding with social relations and being displayed in "social dramas." Unfortunately, he fails to elaborate on how these social dramas actually resolve: apart from the treated individual, the supportive peer group does not at all represent previous problematic social relations, which, therefore, in this context, cannot be restored but, at best, substituted. Moreover, despite my observations that Spiritist practices consist of manifold performative elements, Wiencke ignores the bodily and sensory aspects of healing practices (see Chapter 4).[7]

Theissen (2009) also focuses on practices of cognitive manipulation in Spiritism, particularly within Kardecist psychiatry, but develops a somewhat critical, if not hostile, perspective. As the first non-Brazilian medical anthropologist, she conducted field research at the *Hospital Espírita André Luiz* (HEAL, "Spiritist Hospital André Luiz") in Belo Horizonte (Minas Gerais) to investigate "[...] how religious belief influences professional medical ethics and choices, and the cultural adaptations of bio-medicine in non-western contexts" (Theissen 2009: 1).[8] Unfortunately, she notably reduces her exploration to moral discourse, arguing that the assumption of psychiatric patients being persons who conducted failures in past lives and therapy would have to undergo moral transformation that neglects biological predisposition, social factors, and traumatic experiences (Theissen 2006: 324). Theissen applies a Foucauldian perspective (cf. Foucault 1988a, 1995) on psychiatry as a practice of discipline and displays explicit critique and emotional resistance toward her research field (Theissen 2009: v), presenting a highly biased and lopsided account.[9] She observes social Darwinist, racist, and eugenic attitudes (ibid.: vi), and her report reads like declaring Spiritist psychiatry the religiously masked agent of fascist body politics, social control, and conspiracy of "whitening" the Brazilian population in terms of European values of rationality, order, and progress, sanctioning any deviant behavior. She accuses practices of charity and care as efforts to reproduce unequal social and political conditions by instructing the disadvantaged to work harder on themselves instead of fighting for social justice and structural reforms (Theissen 2009: 21, 196). Accordingly, Spiritist psychiatry would regulate and discipline abnormal behavior and preserve social power relations (ibid.: 213f). Instead of medicalization, Spiritists would morally control lower social classes: "Spiritism represents a discourse of social distinction and justifies the status quo of a high inegalitarian society" (ibid.: 246).

Theissen mentions some examples of Spiritist practices such as *captação*, disobsession, *passe*, and inner reform, but she hardly provides any detailed observation, description, or analysis of these techniques. Instead, she focuses on a few actors, such as the psychiatrist, director of HEAL, and member of AME, Dr. Roberto Lúcio Vieira de Souza, whom she criticizes for only prescribing "psycho-pharmaceutical cocktails" (ibid.: 98), but she does not consider the complementary aspect of psychotropic drug application and Spiritist practices. Without systematically investigating the latter, Theissen draws a somewhat fragmented image of what Spiritist psychiatry is and how spiritual treatment works. Accordingly, without profound accounting, Theissen questions the Spiritists' claim of being scientific and states that their methods and discourses are unprecise, old-fashioned, and even misogynist (ibid.: 31f).[10] Her twisted main argument is that Spiritism has been rejected and even pathologized by secular medicine and mainstream science and that Spiritist science would only reproduce fragments of conventional psychiatric discourse to appear legitimate as a health practice (ibid.: 36). Overall, Theissen develops important insight into Spiritist psychiatry regarding moral implications but also draws questionable conclusions due to methodological disadvantages: she rejects her research field and does not reflect her bias in her interpretation. Instead of participating in distinct practices and engaging with involved agencies, her primary informants belong to the Brazilian anti-psychiatry movement outside HEAL. She does not deliver detailed accounts of practices or refer to interviews with patients and relatives. She, therefore, lacks insight into the therapy process and fails to recognize its potential for personal (spiritual) transformation and the development of patients' agency (see Chapters 3 and 4). Moreover, her critique of Spiritist psychiatry as a national project of social control developed by white elites lacks evidence. Quite the opposite, with their partial autonomy from public health policies and the devotion of volunteers, Spiritist psychiatric hospitals have increasingly become the only remaining spaces of inpatient mental healthcare, attempting to provide sustained medical and spiritual support (cf. Ciello 2013, 2019).

Interestingly, having explored the same institution as Theissen, US-American psychologist Bragdon (2012a,b,c) praises the efficacy of healing practices within Spiritist psychiatry regarding spiritual transformation, personal agency, and new perspectives on life. She proclaims their universal importance and postulates their implementation into US-American psycho-therapy (cf. Bragdon 2004). She proposes investigating the efficacy of Spiritist therapeutic practices to improve healthcare systems worldwide, criticizing contemporary reduction to neuro-biological explanatory models and the exclusive reliance on conventional psychotropic drugs with their serious side effects and lack of significant, sustained improvement (Bragdon 2012a: 10f). To transform mental healthcare toward a more effective and humane model and achieve higher levels of well-being, it would be necessary for physicians to remain open-minded to the range of alternative therapies and integrate them into their current models of biomedical psychiatry. She declares

> Spiritism a unique, safe, and powerful way towards helping people to address chronic mental and physical problems through healing that complements conventional health care. It encourages people to take steps to manifest their highest potential for wisdom, peace, and creativity.
>
> (Bragdon 2012a: 13)

She stresses that "Spiritism not only supports mental health and spiritual growth but does not deplete anyone's bank account. It is not an arm of government or any church. It is wholly supported by private donations" (ibid.: 13). Accordingly, Spiritist practices are community-based grassroots movements available for anybody regardless of religion, race, economic status, gender, or age. Approximately 13,000 Spiritist centers and 50 Spiritist psychiatric hospitals would attend 20–40 million Brazilians and, thus, at least 10% of the Brazilian population. However, Bragdon also stresses their transnational importance:

> More than 45 groups of individuals from the USA, Israel, China, Europe, and Africa have come with me to visit these centers. All are amazed at the resources the centers and hospitals provide and wonder how we might create something similar to benefit them at home. It seems obvious to us that the Spiritist centers and hospitals are giving us a model of integrative health maintenance for physical and mental health. We have nothing like them in the USA or Europe.
>
> (Bragdon 2012a: 13f)

Bragdon provides several translocal case studies to illustrate how mental health issues have been resolved by modifying lifestyle behavior according to Spiritist methods and integrating mediumship training. Even though she admits translation problems regarding the transfer of practices from one cultural context to another, she stresses Kardecism's care resources for Brazilians and non-Brazilians:

> Brazilian healing practitioners represent a new paradigm that encompasses spiritual reality and the effects of evolution over lifetimes as a direct source of illness and wellness. [...] It is time to enhance a cross-cultural exchange. (1) To help Brazilians conduct research, they are involved in focusing on the effectiveness of Spiritist protocols, as well as to evaluate and refine programs for training mediums and healers. (2) To offer students of health care outside of Brazil opportunities to come to Spiritist Healing Centers and Psychiatric Hospitals for further study and training.
>
> (Krippner & Bragdon 2012: 264f)

Bragdon's personal and emotional engagement with Kardecism as a resource for mental healthcare is as evident as Theissen's (2009) rejection of it, and it has been the purpose of this chapter to introduce complementary, opposing, and contradictory perspectives on the intersection and correlation of Spiritism and psychiatry in Brazil. Framed by a related discourse on rationalization and modernization, I have contextualized the emergence of Spiritism in Europe, its implementation in Brazil, and its engagement with mental healthcare within particular medical care systems and their contemporary challenges. Based on my own field research, I will discuss contemporary Spiritist practices, their integration into mental healthcare, and approaches to Healing Cooperation (see Chapter 3) in the following chapters. Addressing the question of how healing practices affect participants, I will further investigate sensory-bodily aspects of human perception and the Aesthetics of Healing in Spiritist mental healthcare (see Chapter 4) before picking up Bragdon's approach and exploring the translocal transfer and transformation of Spiritist healing practices with the example of "Spiritism 2.0" after 200 years of elaboration in 21st-century Germany (see Chapter 5).

Notes

1 Canadian and US-American psychiatrist Dr. Ian Stevenson implemented the Division of Personality Studies at the University of Virginia, USA, that integrated research on paranormal phenomena, including children's memories of previous lives.

2 See https://www.globalhealthrights.org/wp-content/uploads/2013/10/Caracas-Declaration.pdf.

3 See, for example, the International Hearing Voices Network (https://www.hearing-voices.org/).

4 Brazil provides an anthropological goldmine for investigating the "mindful body" (Scheper-Hughes & Lock 1987) at the intersection of individual bodily experience and performance, socio-cultural meaning, symbolism, and body politics framed by political, medical, and media discourse. Scheper-Hughes (1994), as a result of her field research with Brazilian sugarcane workers, develops the concept of the "subversive body" that responds to structural violence with somatic idioms of distress.

  What has struck me most since I first visited Brazil in 2001 is the alleged dialectic between ignorance regarding environmental pollution and pre-occupation with self-care. While I am concerned about not spoiling the environment and becoming irritated with the overall pollution, many of my Brazilian companions do not care. On the beach, they engage in their social and sportive performance and bikini marks but are not disturbed by swimming and sunbathing, surrounded by plastic bottles, cans, straws, and cigarette butts. I wonder if this contradictory engagement with aesthetics is a strategy to cope with an "ugly" reality by performing a beautiful one. It would correspond with Brazilian sociologist DaMatta's approach (1997), which attests to the Brazilian population's tendency to keep "its house clean" while not bothering with the "dirt in the street" as long as it does not affect the individual well-being.

5 I am critical of such culturalism and stereotype generalizations. However, it reveals some aspects of sensory-bodily practices and codes in Brazil that I will investigate in Chapter 4.

6 To some extent, the Brazilian concept of *nervos* corresponds to Kleinman's (1988a,b) investigation of neurasthenia in China as an explanatory model for distress that avoids social stigmatization regarding psychiatric diagnoses.

7 Turner distinguishes two poles of symbols as the minor units of ritual action due to their perceptual qualities. On the one hand, symbols are sets of meaning (signifiés) on a cognitive, perceptual level, but they also act as a perceptible sensory vehicle of experience on a pre-reflective level (Turner 1982: 23).

8 Theissen's statement implies several shortcomings, simplifications, and reductions regarding Kardecism that I intend to clarify. Contrary to an emic self-image, she reduces Spiritist practices to "religious beliefs" without reflecting on the term and its implications. I also disagree with her referring to Brazil as a "non-Western context" and would instead suggest discussing alternative modernities (cf. Gaonkar 2001).

9 Theissen even reflects on these issues but does not analyze their impact on her conclusions.

10 In fact, Theissen's argument is unscientific as she bases her accusations on a single encounter with Spiritist neuroscientist Sergio Felipe de Oliveira's theory on the pineal gland as the location of mediumship capacities (cf. de Oliveira 2009), maybe not being aware of different cultural modes of gender relations.

Chapter 3

Healing Cooperation
Therapeutic Spaces of Brazilian Spiritism

The *Hospital Espírita de Marília* (HEM; Spiristist Hospital of Marília) is located in a somewhat rundown middle-class and semi-residential environment on the top of a hill overlooking the town center of Marília, São Paulo/ Brazil. My first impression upon arrival is the soothing low noise level and relative chilliness inside this simple brick and roughcast building painted in white and blue. I perceive it as a contrast to the hot and noisy environment of a commercial center in one of the hottest regions of Brazil. Entering HEM, the visitor accesses a waiting area in a hallway that connects the public and administrative sections of the hospital with the inpatient wards, separated by locked steel doors. The cold brick benches on either side of the hallway are not very comfortable but help to cool down and relax after coming in from the outside's heat, noise, and busyness. Despite having an appointment to meet the directory of HEM, I wait for almost an hour, flipping through some monthly distributed Spiritist journals and watching staff, patients, and relatives slowly passing by as if to avoid any exertion or bodily engagement. The only annoyances are the continuous announcements and instructions for staff members by shrieking and cracking speakers all over the hospital, which makes me feel displaced to a train station (Figure 3.1).

Finally, Cibele shows up. She works as a psychologist at HEM and is responsible for human resources. She has been my initial contact and now introduces me to Vincente and Bruno. Vincente is the current chairman of HEM's biannually elected Spiritist council, an institutional authority to warrant the Spiritist orientation alongside structural and economic functionality. He has worked here for over 30 years in different functions, and his son Bruno has already been an employed accountant for 4 years. It comes to my awareness that this meeting serves the purpose of a decision regarding the approval or rejection of my project. However, they are very polite and offer the mandatory *cafezinho* ("small cup of coffee") before engaging in a rather philosophical discussion that serves the end of testing my knowledge and eliciting my opinion on Spiritism. They are afraid that I might negatively report on Kardecist practices and stress that in line with Brazilian secular laws, HEM does not provide any religious service but applies a scientifically

DOI: 10.4324/9781032637167-3

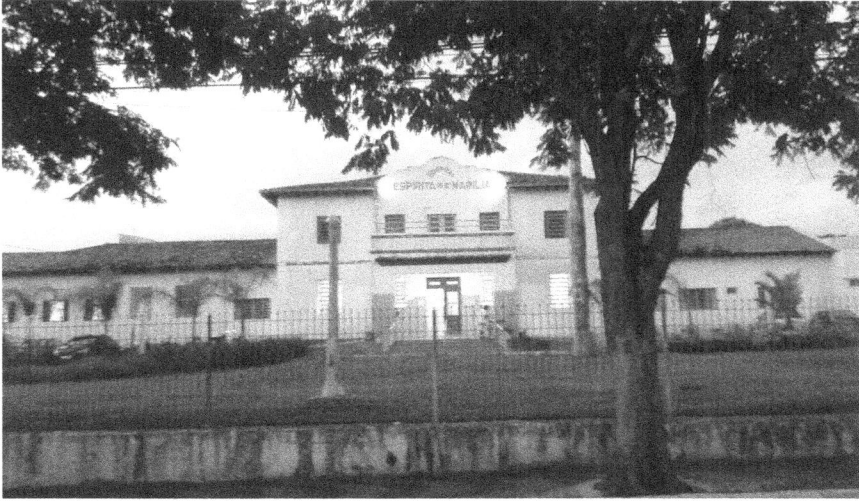

Figure 3.1 Front view of *the Hospital Espírita de Marília* (Photography by HK 2015).

based approach to improve the well-being of the patients. When I mention that I already studied Afro-Brazilian religions and that it is not my aim to evaluate but to describe their practices, they appear to be relieved. They acknowledge my project's potential to inform people abroad about "the truth" of Kardecism and thus shed a good light on them. They grant free access to all areas as long as staff members or Spiritist volunteers accompany me, and the initial insecurities develop toward mutual trust.

As an exemplary environment of Spiritist mental healthcare, in this chapter, I will introduce Marília in the state of São Paulo/Brazil as my research site, focusing on the interconnected institutions of a Spiritist psychiatric hospital and a Kardecist center. I will observe their day-to-day practices (e.g., lectures, study groups, evangelization, fraternal attendance, energetic treatments, mediumship training, and disobsession) and relate them to the narratives of involved individuals. Toward the end of this chapter, I will discuss my observations and perceptions regarding Healing Cooperation as an applicable anthropological model to examine the interrelatedness of (self-)care, providing space for voices crucial for investigating the Aesthetics of Healing in Chapter 4.

Marília

Marília is one of the historic centers of Brazilian Kardecism with a high density of Spiritist institutions, and the *Hospital Espírita de Marília* (HEM) is a psychiatric hospital administered by a committee of local Kardecist associations. Located inland of the relatively wealthy Brazilian Southeastern state of São Paulo, Marília, with its 200,000 inhabitants, constitutes a local economic, commercial, political, educational, cultural, and religious center in an agricultural environment. Until the early 20th century, the area was mainly inhabited by the Indigenous ethnic group of *Coroados*; a hundred years later, no traces of the Indigenous culture exist anymore. From 1900 onward, foreign pioneers from Germany, Italy, Portugal, Japan, and Syria arrived to inhabit and agriculturally develop the remote and climatically extreme arid region. With the international economic coffee peak in 1928, Marília became the final destination of a railway connection to transport products and workers between the inland of São Paulo state and the seaport of Santos and from there to the rest of the world. In the 1930s and during World War II, Marília developed as a center of agriculture, commerce, and industry. By 1938, it held Brazil's first central bus station, with daily buses transporting people from the railway station to the neighboring settlements and farms. In these earlier times, Brazilians related to Marília as one of the centers of Brazilian modernity; in 2015, the railway no longer works, and public bus transportation is insufficient. Due to the relative wealth, most people travel by car or motorbike, but on market days, some visitors arrive by horse, depicting Marília's charming blur of "traditional" rural and "modern" urban life. Entirely fitting the occasional appearance of cowboys in town, Marília stretches around a steep canyon resembling the shape of a horseshoe in a three-partite structure. The Southwest is dominated by institutions and infrastructures of the Federal University of São Paulo State (UNESP). The North is mainly shaped by commerce and middle- to upper-class residential areas, which extend toward a small local airport with two daily flights to and from Campinas. The Southeast is predominated by more impoverished settlements and industrial areas close to the highway connecting the metropolises of Campinas and São Paulo with the interior and the neighboring states. At first sight, these settlements appear as *favelas* ("shanty-towns"), but compared to other cities in Brazil, these suburban environments are less threatening due to relative wealth and sufficient infrastructure. I was able to explore all areas of Marília by bicycle and never felt discomfort apart from the unbearable heat, the sweaty hills, and the intersecting heavy rains, which would transform streets into rivers and finally float as cascades and waterfalls into the canyon, leaving the town and its environment clean and blessed. Empty and decaying buildings and halls, including the former railway station, indicate a certain loss of wealth and national importance, but commerce is still vital, and the number of gas stations, parking lots, shops, and banks allow the impression of a well-structured urban economic center in the geographical periphery of Brazilian modernity. Accordingly, the fact that many beautiful residential family houses from the second half of the 20th century are for sale does not so much reflect the local but a general contemporary economic crisis of Brazil. Marília is still considered a comparably wealthy town, visible not only by the number of private clinics, hotels, bars, and restaurants but also by its clean and structured appearance. People are friendly and helpful, especially toward rare foreign visitors.

The healthcare infrastructure of Marília consists of numerous pharmacies and private clinics, several public health centers, a center for psycho-social assistance (CAPS), a public hospital with a psychiatric emergency unit, a university clinic, and the Kardecist psychiatric hospital HEM, which affiliates with the about twenty Spiritist centers spread all over the town. While most appear to be neighborhood oriented, the *Centro Espírita Luz e Verdade* (CELV, "Spiritist Center of Light and Truth"), with its extraordinary size, substantial public events, and a bookstore/library with several hundred Kardecist books and DVDs, seems to be the headquarter of Kardecism in Marília. Members of CELV founded HEM in 1956 to provide primary mental healthcare with the support of volunteers. These volunteers are members of all social strata of Marília and gather at CELV to learn and discuss Spiritist knowledge. They also engage in charity and community projects, and some focus their dedication on the spiritual support of HEM and their care of psychiatric patients. I followed these volunteers in their daily practices and will introduce some of them throughout the subsequent chapters.

Hospital Espírita de Marília

HEM constitutes the temporary home of up to 250 psychiatric patients within emergency, long-term, and day-clinic wards, subdivided into units according to gender, diagnosis, health plan, and personal resources. A staff of approximately 200 persons and some 50 Spiritist volunteers engage in a complementary therapeutic approach of pharmaceutic, psychotherapeutic, and spiritual treatment. HEM is partly funded by the public Brazilian unitary healthcare system SUS but also offers special accommodation and treatment to patients with a private health plan. These reside in the "Allan Kardec" section, which appears to be a pretty comfortable unit where patients of different ages, genders, and diagnoses mix and interact. The administration of HEM provides three main classifications to distinguish and categorize patients in the SUS wards: "addiction," "psychosis," and "depression." They can interact throughout the day, besides meals and therapeutic interventions such as group or occupational therapies. The only restriction is, with a few exceptions, the segregation of men, women, and adolescents. Employed psychiatrists only spend a few hours a day here since they also affiliate with the public hospital of Marília or run their private clinics. Treatment mainly consists of pharmaceutical and occupational therapy, complemented by efforts to maintain basic psychotherapeutic support, at least for those patients who can afford it. HEM also holds a day clinic for patients with advanced therapy progress and social resources and an asylum for abandoned individuals. The unit for adolescent patients closed earlier in 2015 due to a new federal law generally prohibiting the internalization of minors.

According to my interlocutors within the administration, HEM faces a critical financial situation; particularly, the asylum and SUS units are in a marginal state. Maintenance of services, therefore, has depended on donations and the income of the private health-plan section. Now, a new federal law implementing the Brazilian health policy of deinstitutionalization prohibits mere psychiatric hospitals but tolerates general clinics with psychiatric units. Therefore, upon my arrival in late 2015, the administration of HEM implemented, again with private donations and the personal dedication of volunteers, a surgical unit for two purposes: to raise income through patients with a private health plan and to gain the status of a polyclinic and thus avoid restrictions or even closure by public health officials. As a result, HEM remains one of the few psychiatric clinics in the state of São Paulo that treat patients in acute crisis and grant asylum to individuals who have been ignored by the ambitious Brazilian psychiatry reforms: those who lack any means to take care of themselves, those who do not bear any social resources to be taken care of, and those who are deemed worthless in a cultural environment that stigmatizes mentally disabled and psychiatric patients.

Entering HEM, the visitor passes a reception on the right and a crossing hallway that stretches to the left and right with offices for administration and staff members. On the left, a stairway leads to the second floor with more offices and meeting rooms. Going straight, we pass the waiting area and public bathrooms. A locked iron door separates this public space from the restricted areas, first revealing a simple hall with tables, chairs, and a kiosk with beverages and snacks as a meeting space for patients and their relatives. Three other locked doors lead to the laundry, kitchen, and a blank dining hall with room for 20–30 persons. This is where SUS patients have their four to five daily meals, coming in groups according to their wards and having to finish in 20–30 minutes before the next group arrives. Another locked gate leads to a vast inner courtyard with mango trees full of fruits and shade, benches, a soccer field, and a boccia space. The whole area appears to be in a poor but functional state, and many male patients stay here for hours conversing, smoking cigarettes, and killing time. A tiny carpentry on the left and a big hall on the right with several tables serve as resources for occupational therapy where patients can read, play games, or produce handicraft items, and as an economic resource of HEM, volunteers organize monthly bazaars to sell some of these items. Separated by a wall, this hall extends to an assembly hall that serves occasional theater performances by patients and daily morning lectures by Spiritist volunteers (Figure 3.2).

Crossing the courtyard to the far left, we reach the ward of male patients with psychiatric diagnoses of psychosis, schizophrenia, and depression. They

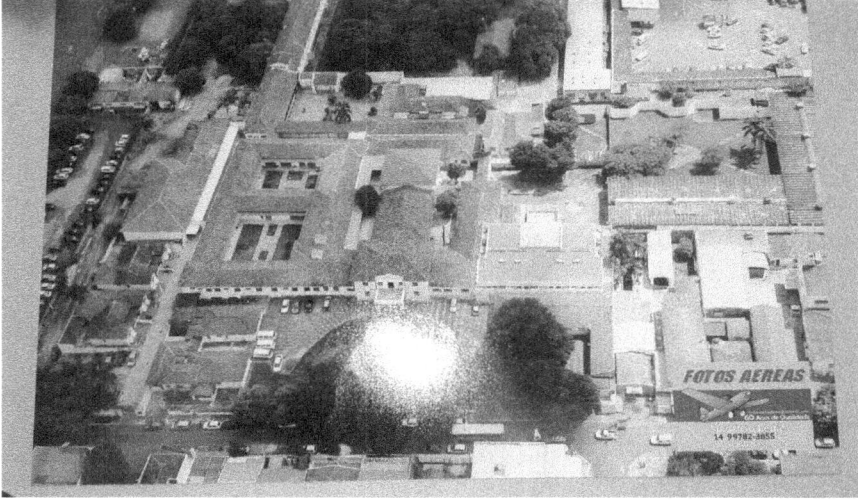

Figure 3.2 Topography of HEM (Photography by HK 2015).

stay here for a maximum of 30 days for acute and mainly pharmaceutic treatment. The ward has several sparse rooms, each with eight iron beds and old mattresses with rough woolen blankets. There is no decoration or space for private belongings. A small room with three-sided glass walls appears to be the nurse's room and a panopticon to observe acute cases and the unit's hallway. Another room serves as a joint facility to watch television or to participate in group therapies with Spiritist volunteers and psychiatrists. I learn that each ward has its fixed team of nurses and cleaning staff but that the psychiatrists, psychologists, social workers, occupational therapists, and Spiritist volunteers move between the units, as does a professional beauty assistant who provides haircuts, pedi-, and manicure. Separated by another locked door but with access to the same courtyard, the unit for male drug-addicted patients resembles the former unit in size and style. Passing another locked iron door, we enter the section of the permanent residents abandoned by their communities and with nowhere else to go. Many are not even diagnosed as psychiatric but as mentally disabled patients. It is a charitable act of the administration of HEM to provide shelter to them as this type of care is neither funded by SUS nor any other official institution. Accordingly, this unit is miserable and permeated by the smell of urine and feces. Even the sleeping rooms are completely tiled to facilitate the cleansing of human excrement. In contrast, a relatively tidy occupation room serves as a space where residents produce handicrafts such as oven cloths or mats, and a remote green and peaceful courtyard segregates them from other patients. This ward leaves me shocked and disgusted, and it will take months until I will be able to return. My disgust relates not only to my sensory experience of an environment I perceive as inhumane but also to the manifest detachment of society from some of its weakest members. Only the Spiritist volunteers care and, in return, receive strong affection and thankfulness.

What a difference and relief it is to pass two more locked iron doors and enter the private health-plan section "Allan Kardec." The two wards are separated according to patients' gender by lockable passages that usually remain open throughout the day. Colonnades surround two neat inner courtyards, patients inhabit single or double bedrooms with private bathrooms, and food is delivered five times daily. There are plenty of benches, couches, armchairs, and tables or shelves with books, games, and even some instruments to provide comfort and distraction. According to Cibele, it always stays full due to its almost spa-like condition and brings extra money from private health insurance or the wealthy families of patients. There is no time limit to the stay of residence, and some patients live here for months or even years as long they or their families pay for it. Whereas patients from Marília dominate the SUS wards, "Allan Kardec" is also frequented by patients from the neighboring towns and areas.

The day clinic is a liminal space between HEM's secluded and public areas. Patients stay here to receive their medication and engage in occupational therapy throughout the day before returning to their families in the afternoon. The unit connects with a huge kitchen where volunteers produce food items for sale to support HEM financially. Leaving it and heading back toward the public parking lot in the front of the hospital, five tiny houses formerly served as residences for staff members but are now inhabited by permanent residents of HEM whom the administration considers partially able to take care of themselves. Social workers support the flat-share inhabitants in organizing daily life and social participation. Three vans parked in front of the hospital take them, and occasionally inpatient groups, to the cinema, for an ice cream, or to participate in other activities to maintain and reestablish contact with the outside world and foster social (re)integration.

Entering the hospital again from the front, but turning right at the big inner courtyard, we pass another locked gate and reach the female SUS section with a smaller yard. It may not be in as good condition as "Allan Kardec," but it seems tidier and has a more relaxed atmosphere than the male SUS section. Another locked iron door leads us to the adolescent ward, but it has been closed and soon will become the before-mentioned surgery ward.

Morning Lectures with *Passe*

Every morning around 8 o'clock, 10–20 volunteers and up to a hundred patients gather in the "theater." It resembles an industrial hall aesthetically, but with its rows of wooden chairs, a few paintings on the wall, and an elevated stage, it becomes a space for patients of all wards to start the day together. It is one of the few occasions where female and male patients can hang out together; some do not miss the chance to flirt and hold hands. However, the majority come to listen to lectures on the Spiritist doctrine provided by one or two volunteers. They communicate lessons on loving and forgiving oneself and others and promote ethical life rules to support personal transformation. Some patients wander around aimlessly and are apparently incapable of intellectually comprehending these messages. Still, according to my Spiritist interlocutors, "it is the spirit that listens," which means that it is not so much about rational understanding but about participating and opening up. Patients and staff members gather and complement each other with a hearty *bom dia* ("good morning") on our way to the assembly hall. A central pathway divides the rows of wooden chairs into two sections meant to separate male from female patients, but neither patients nor staff members seem to care. A vast painting depicting Jesus Christ resurrecting a dead child in its mother's arms serves as a backdrop for the stage that supports a big wooden table with white linen and some chairs around it, a lectern, and a sound system. Pink curtains with silver stars frame the stage and, with a piano and a few spotlights, indicate its alternative use for theater performances and other events (Figure 3.3).

Upon arrival, some patients enthusiastically welcome the volunteers with affection and the accompanying anthropologist with curiosity. Others arrive guided by nurses and will also first salute the volunteers before looking for a seat as close as possible to them. While everybody arrives and looks for their space, meditative music plays for about ten minutes before two middle-aged women enter the stage. One says an opening prayer begging "all the good

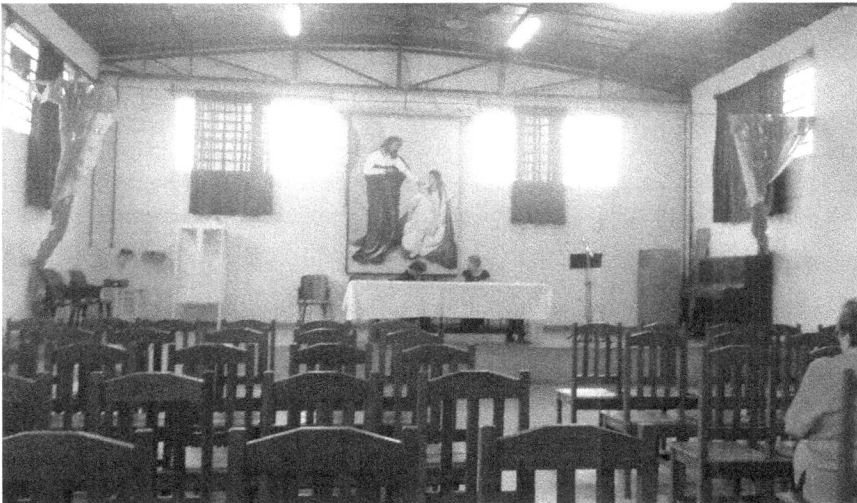

Figure 3.3 HEM's "Theater" (Photography by HK 2015).

spirits" for support and guidance, followed by the other, who discusses aspects of the "Gospel According to Spiritism" by Allan Kardec (2008), addressing the challenge of promoting love, charity, and pardon to oneself and others. They usually speak slowly, quietly, and in an almost slumberous manner for about 30 minutes. Some patients and residents come and go, walking around the hall. Others start a conversation with their neighbors and change seats whenever they feel like meeting or talking to someone else they have spotted. However, this restlessness and skittishness do not seem to disturb anybody, neither the lecturers nor the listeners: everybody seems to be comfortable the way they are, and most participants are tolerant of their fellows' condition without feeling disturbed or distracted. I am convinced many cannot cognitively understand the lecture's content, but they do not seem to bother.

Like all Spiritist gatherings in Marília, the session finishes with the *passe* as a laying-on-hands treatment to fluidically support the *perispirit* of patients and the Lord's prayer as a remedy against spiritual afflictions or disturbances. The lecturer announces the procedure as an energetic treatment for anybody who would accept it. She promotes it as a positive energy provided in the name of Jesus Christ by benevolent spirits through human mediums. Nobody should be afraid since it would not magically or physically manipulate them but instead would work like a transfusion that substitutes negative energies with positive ones and, therefore, supports the patients' capacities to take care of themselves. About ten Spiritist volunteers pass from row to row and stay in front of the patients for about a minute, moving their hands around the recipient's body without touching it. Again, meditative music chimes in the background, and I stay with my eyes shut. Suddenly, I feel a soothing sensation all over my body, and I watch, still with my eyes closed, a kind of spiral or tunnel developing toward a bright light. Before entirely opening up and almost becoming consumed by this feeling, I perceive slight touches on my head and shoulders, which I interpret as a signal that the *passe* has finished. I open my eyes and see that it is Terencio. He moves on to my neighbor, and after ten minutes, the procedure comes to an end as the two speakers finish the session with another thanksgiving prayer to the benevolent spirits and the Lord's prayer, followed by the applause of patients and mutual wishes to have a nice day and God's blessings.

Terencio is a member of the Kardecist administration committee and participates almost daily in the morning lecture to provide *passe* to the patients. He is 74 years old and has worked at HEM for 53 years. He started as a driver and went on with other janitor jobs before, 20 years ago, graduating in law and administration. Since then, he has been the principal accountant for HEM but continued as a Spiritist volunteer, providing *passe*, organizing study groups, and participating in disobsession meetings. The staff of HEM and the Spiritist volunteers respect him as a reliable spiritual adviser, and he constitutes a nodal point of the Kardecist network of Marília and beyond in terms of public relations. He also organizes bazaars and *feijoadas* (public gatherings with a typical Brazilian dish of beans and pork, traditionally served on Saturdays) to raise additional funds for HEM. After one of the morning sessions, we have tea in his office for him to explain the nature of practices:

> I experience it as very positive because many patients never had any religious ties. People live their lives without bothering, and our approach is to provide some knowledge about religion so that upon leaving, they follow a new path instead of sticking to their previous habits. [...] We study the words of Jesus, his parables, and sermons according to the insights of Allan Kardec. He analyzes the parables and discusses what Jesus really wanted to communicate: messages of comfort and hope. Spiritism provides knowledge on the 'why' of suffering, and people stay comfortable with it. They listen to it, and it helps them to cope with their conflicts. They start to think and reflect. They will start to act differently and will develop new perspectives. [...] Our previous actions in this and former lifetimes affect our current life experience, and we have to work on it. Illness, therefore, is not a punishment but a challenge to develop. [...] The practice of *passe* is very important to support this spiritual progress: the medium passes on positive fluids, that is, energy, to another person. [...] It reaches every single cell of the material body but also impacts our spiritual equilibrium and well-being. Moreover, especially in the case of patients with heavy perturbations, we will have to deal with and neutralize spiritual obsessors. The *passe* already helps to neutralize some of the obsessor's forces and to stabilize the patient's equilibrium. It is essential because psychiatric issues are always related to energetic conditions of the *perispirit*. We do not dispense allopathy, for it works on the material body, but by the *passe*, we work with energies. The two approaches are complementary; you must have both.
>
> (Interview 01 Dec. 2015)

Terencio provides a clear-cut image of what Spiritist healing practices are about: they complement conventional psychiatric treatment by adding a spiritual level that (re)distributes agency to patients, reflecting on their experiences, and developing new strategies to cope with them. One central mechanism seems to be the substitution of existent feelings of guilt, failure, shame, and stigma by prospects of forgiveness, hope, self-responsibility, and being part of a "normal" process that everybody has to absolve. Thus, the boundaries of "normal" and "abnormal" behavior and experiences are dissolved, and patients are accepted and integrated as individuals who must actively resolve life challenges instead of being victims of their condition. Based on this conviction, Spiritist volunteers also visit the distinct wards in the afternoon to further discuss with the patients the implications of their experiences.

Evangelization

Once a week in each ward, Spiritist volunteers organize particular one-hour meetings to discuss the spiritual implications of the patients' experiences. Those with a private healthcare plan can even participate in a quiet, comforting atmosphere four afternoons a week. Many experience these sessions as soothing and declare they enjoy listening to and sharing personal insights. I regularly accompany Regina, a Spiritist volunteer and committee member of HEM. We meet about 4 o'clock in the afternoon and head toward the unit "Allan Kardec." Some patients wait at the entrance to welcome and hug her and share chats. We then gather in a comfortable sitting room of the daycare unit with a sofa, a few armchairs, and additional chairs. Regina asks everybody to introduce themselves, and from the moment she mentions that I am here to do research, Elisângela becomes my shadow throughout these meetings. She wants to show and explain everything and make sure that I understand. In return, I teach her some German words, which she will practice until the next meetings. The atmosphere is relaxed and appears more like a roundtable where patients relate shared Spiritist knowledge to their own experiences. Regina starts the conversation with these initiatory remarks:

> Many patients refuse to come here because they think we talk about spirits. However, we do not talk about Spiritism; we talk about self-care, learning how to live and deal with sadness, and resolving our problems. [...] Everybody has to look for what they need.
>
> (Session 18 Nov. 2015)

Specifically, Regina refers to the experience of depression, which many participants are diagnosed with, and they must develop strategies to cope with. The message is that patients are not victims of their condition but are responsible for developing agency. She does not suggest stopping medication but stresses that pills alone will not resolve any problem. Instead, Regina addresses human strategies to deal with negative experiences and needed guidelines. She moves on with the *passe* and declares that it is a positive energy from God. However, she would not force anybody to receive it, and speaking the Lord's prayer would be a vital substitute. A week later, Regina continues with her discourse on depression and introduces the topic of forgiving oneself and others as central to recovery:

> Physical illness can be treated by biomedicine, but there is another aspect: spiritual or emotional illnesses that root deeper and attack our souls in the shape of anxiety or depression. It is about our relationships with people. [...] There is only one remedy for an absolute cure, which goes from inside to outside, not vice versa. [...] It is about forgiving, and it is central to

spiritual progress. Like Jesus said after healing people: "Go and do not sin anymore." [...] It is about inner change, so take care of your inner self and work on your love.

(Session 25 Nov. 2015)

Regina addresses the self-responsibility of patients but adds the aspect of social interaction. She stresses that the attitude toward others impacts human health and well-being. Care and self-care are interconnected, and she asks everybody to start right here, right now, by taking care of their fellow patients. Again, patients can discuss their personal experiences and share examples of how they can support each other before she provides the *passe*.

Evangelization thus resembles a group therapy with a spiritual focus. The reflection and discussion of personal experiences sometimes leave participants crying in (self-)pity and empathy but appear to support them in activating self-healing capacities. Even though each patient's narrative is unique, I want to introduce the example of Elisângela as a representative case study.

In another session in November 2015, the distribution of a little handbill initiates the reflection and discussion of experiences:

Difficulties and trials? They come along with sadness. Many problems on your way? It is disguised help! / You got lost? Do not complain! Stop crying about what puts you down. The science of victory develops from errors. / Weakness does not exist as long as you are not tired of working. There will be no victory when you lose hope. / Injured and insulted? Stick to the rule of love where forgiveness reigns life. The loser will become the winner. / Suffering when it comes finishes with your dreams and peace, but it is a blessing of Heaven for you to know how it is.

(Xavier 1973: 311, translation HK)

The message applies to Regina's previous comments: overcome your self-pity, develop agency, resolve your problems by engaging spiritually, and become a loving and caring being to overcome suffering. Elisângela volunteers to hand out the poem to everybody, reading it out loud and actively participating in the subsequent discussion. To her, the crucial aspect is the first line that states that difficulties and trials will always come along with sadness:

In my case, I was harassed by people close to me, and I brought all this sadness here. However, here I transformed: I talk to God, pray, and praise; this is how I got cured. As in Jesus' sermon on the mountain: I looked and found. [...] God saved me with all the difficulties I had in life, often in the hour of the biggest despair.

(Session 19 Nov. 2015)

Elisângela is a 44-year-old primary school teacher. Her dream has always been to become a veterinary or pediatric doctor and have a family with children to care for. She studied and worked to prevail all her life, but it had not come to be so far. She compensates for it by working with children, which evokes maternal and caring feelings. However, since she was 19 years old, she has suffered from melancholy and sadness after the death of 2 friends. Ever since, she has experienced herself as "too quiet and shy." In 2011, she first went to HEM for psychiatric treatment but returned in October 2015 with a psychiatric diagnosis of bipolar affective disorder. However, she denies her psychiatric diagnosis and stresses the need to live in peace with herself. When I ask her why she is here, she responds:

> I am here because I cannot defend myself against the people who curse and harass me. You know, they tell me to fuck off, and I cry. Therefore, I stay quiet, introspective, and very much for the inside and not for the outside. [...] As they harassed me repeatedly, I started to hate myself. People would not accept me as I am. Therefore, I started to criticize myself, too ... and now that you are talking to me ... one thing is for sure: I did overcome my traumas. [...] I did not like myself because so many people cursed and harassed me.
>
> (Interview 02 Dec. 2015)

She would listen to voices, but when I wondered who would harass her, she only answered that she could not reveal: "I came here to overcome my traumas and the pain – physical pain and pain of the soul – as I said already in the meetings" (Interview 02 Dec. 2015). With "meetings," Elisângela refers to the evangelization sessions with Regina. Within these sessions, she gradually reveals that those who harass her are obsessing spirits she cannot control. She believes that her friends' deaths were partly her responsibility because she foresaw their deaths but did not warn them. She is convinced she is a medium because she would see things, and then these things would happen. She further believes that she must help others to develop and understand her mediumship as a gift of God, which, once received, she has to use. When I ask her what mediumship and the related practice of *passe* would mean to her, Elisângela responds: "It is about helping and developing. [...] It is about love, which is in me, and this love goes to the person who receives. [...] It is a transmission of love, the strongest energy existing" (Interview 02 Dec. 2015).

Elisângela's narrative reflects distinct aspects of Spiritist mental health-care. On the one hand, she takes the evangelization sessions seriously and applies the task of caring for others as a means of self-care. It also reveals how in Spiritist mental healthcare, afflicting experiences are reinterpreted: despite being diagnosed with a bipolar affective disturbance, her main concern was about these "people who would harass" her and her alleged presentiment of the friends' death, which seems to be at least one causing factor of her condition. In Spiritist terms, she can relate these experiences to the explanatory models of obsession and mediumship instead of being an organic defect. It helps her cope with her experiences, and she wants to engage with a Spiritist center to explore it further. As she has revealed throughout our conversations, volunteer Regina serves her as an idol.

Regina is about 75 years old, a widow, a mother of 5, and a retired teacher. She complains that so many people, when commenting on Spiritism, would talk about summoning spirits or magical healing and not what Kardecism really is about: self-healing in terms of dealing with sadness and resolving related personal problems, and evangelization is about love and attention toward others. However, she would not have engaged in this practice for over fifteen years if it would have only been for the sake of the patients:

> I believe that working here is an experience you cannot have anywhere else. When I started here many years ago, there was a friend of ours who was really studied and ahead of us all, and I gave lessons to the patients and went to him and told him: 'I do not like it because I am a teacher and I usually see fast results. Here, I do not! Nothing happens! Nothing is moving forward.' So, he said: 'Why do you think you are here because of them? You are here because of yourself: you need this experience!'
>
> (Interview 07 Jan. 2016)

Regina is of a Catholic background and was a single child. Out of all of her family ties, she especially talks about her father with intense affection. She declares that she grew up fearing spirits and the dark as she would "sense things." From her current perspective, she believes she has already been a medium since the age of twelve when she suffered from insomnia, sadness, and being a reticent child. After Regina married and her first daughter was six months old, her father died of a heart attack at a young age. Later, when she was in her early thirties and pregnant with her second child, some troubling experiences would start to haunt her:

> I always stayed tired, as it is normal for a woman after the second month. Every night at eight p.m., I wanted to go to bed, and my husband would have to accompany me, or I had to sleep in the living room, crashing in front of the TV. Why? I was afraid to stay alone in the bedroom because this phenomenon only appeared when I was on my own. [...] Listening to this voice right in my ear, like an echo of these microphones turned on too loud. This voice would always repeat the same thing: 'My daughter, I love you! I love you a lot, my daughter!' [...] And it left me with fear, I was freaking out, scared. Imagine the situation: my husband would have to go to bed without being tired, or I would stay in the living room because I

was scared of this voice. This phenomenon would repeat several times, the voice always telling me the same thing until, one night, I dared to ask: 'Dad, what do you want from me? Tell me, Dad!' There was no answer but 'my daughter, I love you.' It could not go on like this – so what should I do? I tell you, the only way was to turn to Kardecism because I was terrified.

(Interview 07 Jan. 2016)

Just like Elisângela, Regina had some extraordinary experiences that manifested in listening to voices and connected to the death of loved ones. These experiences could have been easily identified as hallucinations in combination with stress resulting from personal loss and, therefore, as a psychiatric diagnosis of depression and/or psychosis, as was the case with Elisângela. Regina's fate was different: her mother contacted Manoel Saad, one of the founders of HEM and president of CELV at that time. He lived in the same neighborhood and was considered a medium capable of resolving such spiritual issues. Regina does not remember how he did it, but she recalls a mediumship session where a medium would incorporate her father to be instructed on his harmful behavior before being accompanied to "another place" by two guiding spirits. Afterward, Saad would inform her that she is a medium and must work on her ability. Since then, Regina has frequented CELV and participated in study groups whenever possible. To her delight, her husband also turned out to be interested in Kardecism, and they would practice together, which happened to be the best time in her life. She mentions that he was ten years older than her and "the kind of a husband who is more like a father," but in the same breath, she complains that some health issues would occur whenever something was right in her life. Accordingly, some years after the episode with her father, her husband, who was only 50 years old, turned seriously ill and died at the age of 60. Now, she would listen to his voice at night, although in a much more peaceful way than her father's. She does not reveal many details but assures that after this experience, and with all the problems of a single mother with five children, she owes her balance to Kardecism. Especially after retiring, she has spent much time in study groups and tried to further develop her alleged mediumship skills in special training groups. Therefore, besides evangelizing the patients and supporting the administration of HEM, she also participates as a medium in William's disobsession group once a week.

Disobsession

William is a key informant for my understanding of Spiritist mental healthcare. Like Regina, he provides evangelization sessions for the patients of HEM. Being a former member of HEM's administration, he is very determined about the importance of evangelization for the patients. Even though he stresses the importance of the patient's free will to participate, in his opinion, the administration and staff of HEM should engage more in encouraging them; spiritual aspects would have to be taken more seriously. He says evangelization is not just a practice of having patients reflect on their condition; even if they could not cognitively absorb the given information, the obsessors, deranging spiritual agents, would listen and learn about their misbehavior. Therefore, William also promotes disobsession as another spiritual practice to treat afflicted and afflicting spirits. He describes it as crucial to simultaneously treat patients and the obsessors with the help of human mediums. According to him, it works like a "gentle exorcism" and is performed in weekly one-hour meetings of groups of eight to twenty persons. Various groups of volunteers conduct about 20 different disobsession meetings every week at HEM. Patients do not participate because having psychiatric patients engage in mediumship practices is prohibited by law. Another reason is that most Spiritists also deem it dangerous for unprepared people to participate; it could negatively affect them and disturb "the vibration" of the session. Yet another reason is that patients should work on themselves and not take obsessing spirits as an excuse for their behavior and experience. Therefore, the sessions mainly aim at engaging with afflicting spirits in the orbit of HEM. These can be evil spirits who want to disturb the spiritual work or spirits that affect certain patients who are sometimes even identified. However, the focus is not on the patients but on treating these spirits so that they stop their misbehavior and experience support and healing themselves.

A disobsession team consists of mediums, assistants, and an organizing chairperson. They sit around a table in a plain, darkened room without visual distractions. Some books, papers, pens, and a jug of water are the only items on the table, and one may spot a clock or a picture of some Spiritist authority on the wall. The chairperson decides who will perform which task according to a rotation system. One opens the session with an improvised supplication prayer, asking God, Jesus, and benevolent spiritual guides for support. Others recite and discuss Spiritist literature extracts before somebody else recites the Lord's Prayer. Throughout the prayer, another group member extinguishes all the lights and closes the last open windows and curtains to avoid any distractions from the outside. Participants then remain silent, and some seem to concentrate on something within them, most of them with their heads in their hands as if to not hitting the table. Sometimes, participants even fall asleep, and I remember staying unconscious on more than one occasion, not recapturing what had happened during the session. It is the moment that mediums start to perceive the surrounding spirits with all their senses: some see, some hear, some smell, feel, or even taste them, and will then communicate what they perceive. Most participants stay with their eyes closed and will listen to the voice of a medium transmitting alleged messages from a discarnate spirit who suffers from anger, fear, sadness, despair, and confusion and who is considered responsible for some patients' or participants' afflictions in terms of obsession. One or two assistants then perform the actual disobsession that follows a specific pattern. Through the mediums, they converse with the spirits, exploring their condition of death and after-life experiences. They discuss the harmful effects of the spirits' behavior and finally offer care facilities in a hospital on a higher spiritual level, provided by benevolent "spirits of light." These spirits are supposedly always around, supporting the session, taking care of the afflicted and afflicting spirits, and sometimes communicating specific requirements or advice through a medium. Once, after a session, I wondered why these spirits would need our engagement; why would they not resolve all the issues within their spiritual dimension? The answer was that the obsessors were still tied to an energetic level attuning to the material world and, therefore, it would need a bridge from one level to the other. Those participants who stay quiet or fall unconscious throughout the procedure would donate and provide the energy required to lift them. After treating three to five cases, some assistants provide *passe* to everybody, and the same person who spoke a prayer in the beginning now recites an improvised thanksgiving and the Lord's prayer. The water on the table is now considered "fluidized" with positive energies, and everybody consumes a cup of it to internalize the healing spiritual forces.

To provide a livelier idea of the procedure and the conversation between spirits and humans, I am illustrating a session on 24 November 2015. At precisely 5 o'clock in the afternoon, right after his evangelization reunion with patients, William meets Regina, three other men, and five other women in a plain room of the former daycare unit of HEM. The worn-down white walls do not offer any decoration, and the room only consists of a large table with some chairs around and a jug of water. The windows are shut and darkened, and only a few light beams and distorted sounds from the nearby street find their way through cracks and holes. After chatting about future events, Adriana reads a text from Kardec's "Gospel According to Spiritism," focusing on spiritual influences and the power to resist temptation. It takes about five minutes, and the message is that negative thoughts derive from moral imperfection, an external force, or both. All individuals are responsible for thinking positively and fending off these negative influences. The most potent weapons against all evil would be to turn to God and the guiding spirits, pray, and avoid habits of pride, vanity, or egotism. Participants discuss the text, and William comments that he has experienced it as uplifting because it produces positive thoughts.

He then decides who is to perform which role today. Four female mediums are present (Regina, Rosa, Luciana, and Sara). Adriana will continue to be responsible for lectures and prayers, and the other men (Vincente, Osvaldo, and Eduardo) will perform the *passe*. William and Sonia will communicate with the spirits incorporated by the mediums. Sonia locks the door and turns off the light, leaving the room just dimly illuminated, while Adriana speaks an improvised prayer:

> Lord Jesus, our master and patron, protect this group so that it will be valuable for your work. Let us take the necessary steps to support the spiritual world and this house in your hands to help those who come here because they need orientation, support, and love. Please guide and help us, who are all at your disposition.

Then she continues with the Lord's prayer, and even though this interval does not take longer than two minutes, the atmosphere in the room has completely changed: there is absolute silence except for some street noise and birds' songs from outside. They appear to be very far and unreal. All participants have their eyes closed, and most put at least one hand on their forehead to support it against sudden heaviness and tiredness or to protect their eyes from distraction. It is 5:15 pm, and spirits arrive as if there has been an exact appointment. Some participants start to yawn or shiver, and I feel increasing pressure and heaviness on my shoulders without being able to identify the cause. After a minute of total silence, Regina complains she feels some "challenging fluids" around and can hardly breathe. William asks her to stay calm and to breathe, but she becomes increasingly agitated and starts to yell, cry, curse, and whine. From what I understand, and some participants agree afterward, she is incorporating the spirit of someone who died suffocated by mud in a landslide or mining accident. I right away think of Mariana,[1] but it is not further discussed. The spirit reveals that he[2] pursues solid spiritual ties with one of HEM's patients but does not clarify the quality of their relationship. The following fifteen-minute conversation between William and the spirit incorporated in Regina illustrates that any alleged patient–spirit relationship is of no interest here, but that disobsession aims at helping afflicting spirits and, thus, if anything, only indirectly the afflicted persons. It is not about identifying culprits and victims but discussing the self-responsibility for spiritual progress.

Initially, the spirit reacts upset about being "brought here" and complains about being unable to breathe. William tries to calm him down, but the spirit keeps crying and yelling that he wants to return to where he was because nobody could help him. William insists that we are here to help him and that there are "good friends" around; if he would accept this support, he would soon feel relief. This contest continues for several minutes until the spirit becomes less agitated and medium Regina breathes more calmly. Still, the spirit insists that he would have to return to "help the others," but William suggests that he first should take care of himself and that his misbehavior would also affect others. He tries to gain more information about the circumstances of the death, but the spirit whines: "I do not want to remember this past anymore. So many people were lost and got dragged further and further away. There was no light, and I cannot reveal more of this past because they don't let me." William repeats that the spirit first has to take care of himself before being able to care for others who would drag him down instead of allowing him to progress. His behavior would harm himself and others, and he should accept the support of those who want to help him. As the spirit reluctantly gives in, William plays his trump card, mentioning the presence of a guardian angel that the spirit identifies as a companion throughout past lifetimes and agrees to follow him to the "hospital on the spiritual plane."

There is silence for a few seconds before Regina mentions that she still lacks air. It hints that mediums do not just "imagine" or cognitively receive a message but sensory experience and embody this information (see Chapter 4). William tells her that she will soon recover and asks if there is more to say or if any other suffering individual would need attention. Medium Rosa immediately bursts out: "Suffering, suffering... hm ... you make me suffer! What is this? Why do I have to stay in line over here all this time? I will not wait one more minute; I want to be attended now!" From a performative perspective and personal experience, I associate this communication as a metacommentary on healthcare within SUS, where people wait hours without being attended to. Keeping this aspect of hospital mimicry in mind, I interpret the whole session as the performance of a spiritual ambulance. As in any other emergency ambulance, the more severe cases receive treatment first. Accordingly, toward the end of the session, the issues become smoother and "treatment" faster: one spirit complains about how lame this meeting is and asks for some *cachaça* to start the party. Another seems to be a vengeful spirit who enjoys hiding and watching others suffer. The last spirit to appear is a woman of alleged Afro-Brazilian descent who complains that upon death, she was abandoned because she was black and poor. I perceive it as another metacommentary on the Brazilian healthcare system regarding social and racial inequalities in Brazil. William engages in a friendly conversation with her regarding spirituality and health. Commenting on her affiliation with Afro-Brazilian religions, he confirms that she has been on the right track but now will have to take a further step to develop spiritually before reincarnating and having all the support she needs. She leaves gratefully (Session 24 Nov. 2015).

My interpretation of disobsession as hospital mimicry is not meant pejorative but refers to its performative character. It applies to Xavier's elaborations on a "hospital on the spiritual level" (see Chapter 2). The declared aim is to treat people with love (incarnate and discarnate), as is the official slogan of HEM. The disobsession team tries to locate the spirits' afflictions in space and time by exploring when, where, and under which circumstances they died. Then they inform them that they only died materially but that life goes on and that they have to cope with staying without a material body and resolve some spiritual issues before reincarnating again. Like in the evangelization meetings, the main topic is self-responsibility: instead of caring for others, spirits first would have to take care of themselves. Instead of feeling guilty or accusing others, they must experience and practice love. At that point of spirit-human interaction, orienteers always mention a guardian angel or beloved deceased person waiting to welcome, and from one moment to another, the situation switches: the spirit decides to cope.

At 5:50 p.m., William asks if everybody is all right, and Regina mentions feeling exhausted. William promises that soon she will feel better, and the three men perform *passe* on everybody in total silence. It takes about five minutes, and suddenly, I can hear the noises of the street, some birds and dogs, and a radio or television in the background again. It feels like coming back from another dimension. After William says a prayer that very much resembles the initial prayer of Adriana and finishes with the Lord's prayer, there is a brief conversation about what had happened, and many communicate how great this treatment was with all the spirits around. Sometimes, cases of participants and their "accompanying spirits" also play a role in disobsession meetings. Regina's example suggests that engaging here also helps her to deal with "her" spirits. I conclude that participants do not solely care for others but also for themselves, negotiating human–spirit interactions and using their personal experiences as templates to help others.

Centro Espírita Luz e Verdade

Many Spiritist volunteers at HEM also frequent the CELV ("Spiritist Center of Light and Truth"), a two-story complex a few blocks from HEM. It consists of a vast hall fitting over a 100 visitors and 12 smaller rooms for weekly study groups, mediumship sessions, and charitable activities. In addition to donations and income from its bookstore, members help to financially maintain CELV and HEM by selling handmade bakery products and organizing flea markets for second-hand clothing and furniture items. A significant part of financial income is redistributed to charity projects: CELV provides 150 baskets of staple foods to indigent families of Marília every month and up to 600 bowls of free soup every Sunday. Besides these basic material forms of care, practices of fraternal care, study, and mediumship training serve as spiritual strategies to support people in need. Since 2007, César, the son of the co-founder of HEM Manoel Saad, has been the president of CELV, coordinating various activities and providing weekly lectures. He is 60 years old and works as an electrical engineer. He stresses that the continuity of care for over 60 years is due to both spiritual and human efforts, since in 1936, a "guiding spirit" in a mediumship session demanded to engage psychiatric patients with spiritual treatment, laying the foundation of HEM. He does not perceive Spiritism as a religious practice that would bedazzle people in a local context with a charismatic leader but as stimulation of human progress deriving from the spiritual world. Neither does he consider it a Brazilian practice but envisions the global redistribution of Spiritism, not just offering explanatory models for afflicting experiences but also providing guidelines for resolving them (Figure 3.4).

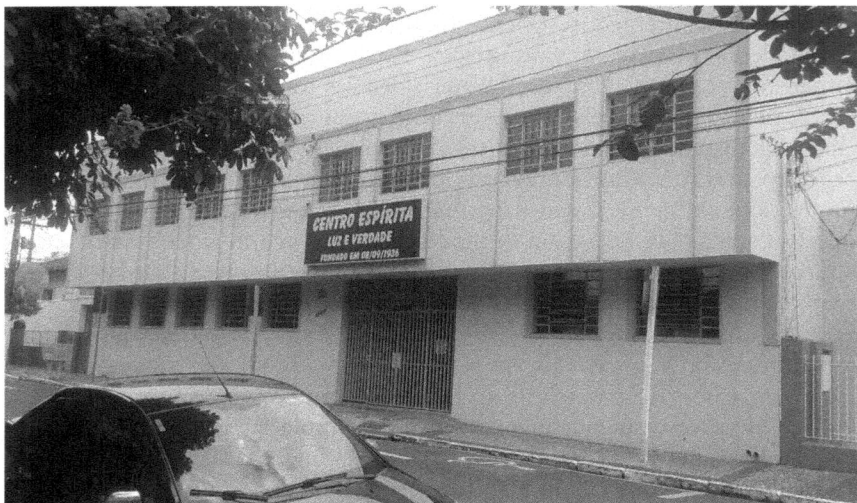

Figure 3.4 Front view of the *Centro Espírita Luz e Verdade* (Photography by HK 2015).

Fraternal Care

CELV offers free fraternal care five nights a week for people in acute social, emotional, mental, or spiritual distress. Some clients report unusual perceptions like hearing voices or seeing "things" that scare them. Their experiences are often rejected as unreal, crazy, or even demonic by their social and religious environments, and feeling desperate and left alone, they come to CELV as a last resort of hope for support. Upon arrival, volunteers hand out numbers and direct them to a waiting room. According to the sequence of numbers, they are called in to talk about their issues with other specially trained volunteers. A disobsession meeting in another room works with obsessing spirits and provides short psychographic messages for the clients. As in HEM, clients do not participate but reflect on their problems relating to the psychographic message and discuss it with the orienteers. After about half an hour of conversation, the client receives a *passe* from another volunteer and is requested to attend a lecture at least once a week and receive a *passe* for the next two months.[3]

The first time I participate in this treatment, I stay with the orienteers. Before the actual treatment occurs, they read and discuss a chapter of Kardec's "Gospel According to Spiritism" for about half an hour. Somebody speaks the Lord's prayer, and then the group decides which orienteer will attend which client. I accompany Melissa to meet Janina in a private small room for a 40-minute conversation; she will be our only client today. Janina is in tears and complains about domestic problems: her marriage would not work out anymore as her husband's wealthy family would not accept her due to her marginal economic and social status. Even though they would love each other, she could not bear the situation anymore and moved out, leaving her daughter behind and feeling depressed. Now, she is looking for a way to return to her family and suggests a Spiritist explanatory model: she might be a medium and too sensitive so that she would be overreactive. Melissa listens for a while and asks questions to understand her situation better. Then, to my surprise, she does not encourage Janina to sit down with her husband to resolve their problems or to explore her mediumship – which, in her opinion, is Janina's attempt to deal with the situation without having to face the "real" problem. On the contrary, Melissa tries to convince her to divorce:

> It does not do you any good. You know that you will feel bad. You must stand your ground. [...] You must leave them doing their thing, and you do your thing. The question is: where do you want to get? [...] Why do you allow yourself to suffer like this? [...] You must be responsible for yourself, and you should not stay in this sadness, regretting that it is over now; you should explore why it happened and what you can learn from it.
> (Session 03 Dec. 2015)

Melissa does not mention any spiritual or mediumistic explanatory models but wants to strengthen Janina as a person, imposing on her the ideal of self-responsibility instead of marital and maternal responsibilities. She suggests that Janina should turn to God by studying Spiritism and discovering what is best for her. In that instance, her personal psychographic message is handed in.[4] Melissa and Janina engage in a discussion over it that leaves Janina crying and finally giving in to everything Melissa says. I perceive it as a radical and unilateral approach, avoiding any possibility of a reunion with the family, but Melissa is convinced that this woman must leave her past behind and concentrate on her present and future. Afterward, I question her "intuitive" spiritual approach that mirrors her background as a relatively independent woman who married and lived for years in Germany, which may not quite apply to others here. Our controversy on this topic became the base for a friendship relationship and a profound debate on what Spiritist healing practices are about and where they could or should not intervene. She declares that this interaction has no rules besides applying Spiritist knowledge and following intuition. When I ask her why she is participating in this kind of practice, she responds:

> I like to help others, and it helps me, too. It makes me feel good and provides relief. For everything around me, I try to reflect on my own life, which helps me be more responsible toward myself and others. It calms me down. I find ways to keep my balance because I have to prepare to give the best attention possible to people mentally. At the same time, it helps me! [...] I learned to reflect on my own experiences. I am asking them why

they think they feel this or that and why they are reacting the way they are. It is for them to reflect, but I must also explain the energetic aspect and the nature of spirits around us. [...] I study to help others and myself. In the first place, I am dealing with myself, studying, and trying to evolve.

(Interview 24 Jan. 2016)

Melissa's statement strengthens my conviction that Spiritist healing practices integrate (self-)care in a way that one's problematic issues will be resolved by supporting others. It is about the agency on both sides: Melissa suggests that Janina acts self-responsibly and actively engages with her problems, and at the same time, she experiences empowerment herself, "bringing out the best in me." Her efforts enhance her self-reflection abilities to make "sense" of her existence. A week later, I witness a somewhat different and complicated case of fraternal care: usually, clients only engage in one introductory conversation before participating in the evangelization process of eight successive weekly lectures with subsequent *passe* and the related consumption of fluidized water. However, in the case of Sabrina, a second conversation has been implemented before directing her to further studies. This time, I accompany Sylvia, and she informs me about her encounter the previous week:

Came that girl, being Pentecostal and suffering a lot. We worked a lot, but she was so devastated that we would need another session. She will not receive another message, but we must give her more orientation. We want to direct her toward the doctrine to be able to help herself, but she is scared. Her whole social environment is of Pentecostal denomination and neglects Spiritism. Therefore, she is trapped in seeking help here without anybody in her community knowing she is doing so.

(Session 10 Dec. 2015)

To comfort her, Sylvia starts the appointment by praying for Jesus to ask for his support and only mentions "the spiritual guides" in a side sentence. She continues with the Lord's prayer, and Sabrina joins in. I learn that for years, Sabrina has perceived "strange things" in her house, listening to voices and feeling the presence of somebody. For over 20 years, it has left her restless and negatively affected her health and social relations. The previous week, her experiences had already been identified as mediumship to be trained, but in her environment, she could not even address it once it would be recognized as a demonic influence. Accordingly, Sylvia suggests that Sabrina study Spiritism, train her mediumship, and, if necessary, leave her social environment once she can receive all social support over here (Session 10 Dec. 2015).

This case is totally different from Janina's, who came with the idea that she might be a medium as an explanatory model or even an excuse for her experience. Sabrina is suffering from extraordinary experiences, which, in psychiatric terms, would direct toward psychotic delusions or hallucinations. However, seeking psychological or psychiatric treatment is expensive for working-class members like her and would result in further social stigmatization. She cannot communicate her experiences within her community as people would interpret them as demonic possession and, in the worst case, exclude or extradite her to exorcist practices. In Spiritism, she finds explanatory models (mediumship and obsession) that neither stigmatize nor exclude her. On the contrary, she is invited to participate in a group of individuals with similar experiences and to explore and develop her unusual sensory perceptions. Besides offering an explanatory model for Sabrina's experience that obviates hospitalization and/or stigmatization, Sylvia stresses aspects of self-responsibility and agency and the possibility of recovery by engaging in the "right" therapy. She returns to Sabrina's spiritual message delivered by the mediumistic group the previous week and reads it out loud for her to reflect on it one more time:

> Welcome to this fraternal care. In the first place, you deserve congratulations for the fact that you chose this house to receive help – to help yourself and those around you. It proves your will to develop, and we will help and support you wherever necessary. The words and orientation you received where you had been before are not good for your health. You must transform that energy to become something beautiful. It is about forgiving and turning toward the work for the good. Master Jesus will guide [...]. Look for your own way of development that links to past lives. Ask yourself why is it that these spirits are harassing you. See it as a test in your actual life. There are some bills to be paid, but this is not the core of it. It is the belief and the wish for change that will make a difference in your life – for you to stay happier and live in peace and harmony.
>
> (Session 10 Dec. 2015)

After knowing Sabrina's narrative, I am surprised at how accurate this message is. I am convinced that there is no trick or "secret communication" between the participants of orientation and disobsession groups. Anyway, I do not want to guess; I observe that it helps Sabrina relax, settle down, and agree to Sylvia's proposal to participate in the eight-week treatment of lectures and *passe*. However, I only see her again twice at CELV, and a year later, Sylvia admits that she lost track of her. She concludes: "We can only offer what we can give, and she knows about the shit she is in but does not know how to get out of it."

Other clients, including former patients of HEM, regularly frequent CELV and experience consolation and recovery by participating in lectures and study groups, practicing charity, and changing their daily routines – in brief, developing a Spiritist habitus. Due to its long-term orientation, I could not follow up on the entire transformational processes of my research partners, but Ana-Paula, a former patient of HEM and a current member of CELV, shared her narrative with me. She is in her late 40s and works as a clerk with the public healthcare administration of Marília. She is of a Catholic background, married, has two children, and lives with her family in their own house. In 2013, "out of the blue and for no reason," she suffered from heavy depression. She could not take care of herself anymore, and her family finally decided to hospitalize her in the private health-plan unit "Allan Kardec" of HEM. In addition to medical treatment and occupation therapy, she attended Spiritist lectures and evangelization meetings. For the first time, Ana-Paula would hear about reincarnation, karma, and obsession. According to her, pharmaceutical and psychotherapeutic treatment did not provide relief, but with time, the daily lectures, discussions, and *passe* experiences did so. Even though she has never had any ties to Spiritism before, she and her family started considering the explanatory model that her affliction might be due to spiritual obsession. After a few months with only gradual pharmaceutical therapy success, she was granted leaving HEM once a week to attend the fraternal care and eight-week treatment at CELV. Right away, mediums and orienteers confirmed the influence of an obsessing spirit. Ana-Paula learned that it would be her responsibility to change her situation but that she would receive support from the spiritual guides and the Spiritist volunteers. For the subsequent eight weeks, she attended the one-hour lectures on Spiritist doctrine, received the *passe*, and consumed the fluidized water. She started to read Spiritist literature and gradually recovered, still taking her medication. At some point, she was released from HEM and returned home, but after a few weeks experienced a relapse. She repeated the eight-week treatment twice, but only when she started attending study groups and participating in charity activities would she experience sustained relief. Now, she feels "new-born," and the attending psychiatrist, a Spiritist herself, progressively reduces her medication. Ana-Paula has started to work again but continues to participate in the lectures and other activities of CELV (Interview 15 Nov. 2015). Her case illuminates how Spiritism does not promise permanent recovery but sustained relief by continuous engagement with Spiritist practices and a re-orientation of life conduct by studying Spiritist knowledge.

Lectures and Study Groups

CELV organizes daily public lectures on the Kardecist doctrine, provided by speakers from a broader translocal network of agencies and institutions. In form, structure, and content, they resemble Spiritist lectures all over the country and, as far as I can relate, around the world: selected speakers pick a particular life aspect or topic and discuss it according to their life experience and personal approach to Spiritism. Different from HEM, lectures can take up to 90 minutes. Participants arrive at CELV and write their names and those they pledge spiritual support for in a textbook. They might pick up some leaflets with excerpts of Kardecist literature to read and reflect on before the lecture begins. Others stay praying or quietly talking to their fellowmen. Throughout the lectures, the audience remains relatively silent and attentive. Some seem to look for visual distraction but do not find any decoration apart from posters informing about Spiritist activities and sometimes digital projections concomitant to the lecture. Afterward, participants line up in front of a secluded room to receive a *passe* by volunteers. According to the number of listeners, this procedure can take another hour and requires patience to wait for everybody's turn, and interlocutors argue that waiting in patience and devotion allows the "higher spirits" to "work" on everybody in spiritual and energetic terms. After the *passe*, participants receive a cup of "spiritually energized" water to consume (Figure 3.5).

Following this eight-week program and before engaging in study groups that focus on specific topics (e.g., mediumship and health), CELV offers three subsequent courses of the *Estudo Sistematizado da Doutrina Espírita* (ESDE; "Systematic Study of the Spiritist Doctrine"), each taking about half a year. CELV distributes textbooks to warrant a systematically structured study progress throughout the weekly one-hour seminars. I attended an initial course named *Conhecendo o Espiritismo* ("Getting to know Spiritism") directed by Silvia. She is 58 years old, married, and recently became a grandmother. She was raised Catholic but declares that she has always been more interested in "science." When she was 42 years old, she suffered from "severe depression." Parallel to psychotherapy, she started to read Spiritist literature and became

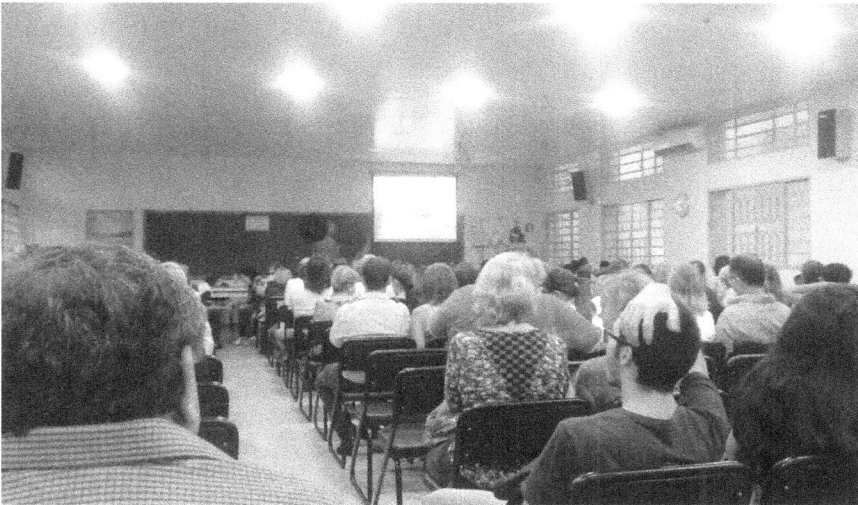

Figure 3.5 CELV's Lectures Hall (Photography by HK 2015).

interested in the topic of mediumship. After studying the books of Kardec, she was convinced that in opposition to Catholicism, Kardecism would provide a scientifically coherent framework of spiritual experiences. She started to engage with several study groups, and soon, one of her instructors invited her to become an orienteer of fraternal care. After a few months, the chairperson of her group would ask her to participate in the disobsession meetings to transmit psychographic messages. She thought it was all a hoax until she wrote down her first message, which supposedly came to her mind intuitively, and all her peers would praise it as a "very nice message." Encouraged by this positive response, she would continue doing so and read Kardec's book on a daily basis to prevent her own thoughts and feelings from infiltrating the spiritual messages. At some point, she would start to produce messages that had nothing to do with what she had read before, and this was the point that she allowed "her intuition to speak." However, after many years of practice, she is still insecure about what are her thoughts and feelings and what comes "from beyond" (Interview 08 Jan. 2016).

Silvia's ESDE course prepares participants to enter a similar path of spiritual progress where they learn to (re)interpret their experiences, organized and structured alongside the textbook, synthesizing various Spiritist authors' works. As with any other Spiritist meeting, the session begins with a prayer for spiritual support and ends with a thanksgiving prayer, the Lord's prayer, and a *passe* provided by Silvia. She encourages participants to improvise prayers by listening to an inner voice before they read paragraphs of the textbook that Silvia then discusses in relation to participants' personal experiences. She provides a framework where individuals can reinterpret their experiences and do so in a way that they acknowledge their agency.

Care and Self-Care

The previous vignettes and case studies reveal the healing cooperation of Spiritist and psychiatric institutions. Cushioning the shortcomings of the Brazilian deinstitutionalization policy (see Chapter 2), Spiritist volunteers complement mental healthcare by initiating and supporting the self-reflection and agency of patients. Iotti, one of HEM's psychologists, is convinced that the Brazilian psychiatry reform bears some progress and that patients should remain within their communities for social support, family networks, and an environment they are accustomed to. However, she declares it a utopia as further political efforts toward social assistance and destigmatization of psychiatric diagnoses would have to come up. According to her, treatment at HEM would not differ much from other mental healthcare institutions apart from the Spiritist approach. She declares that at HEM, weekly supervision of psychiatrists, medical doctors, nurses, psychologists, and occupational therapists serves the interdisciplinary discussion of patients' cases, including spiritual aspects. Spiritism has never been a topic to her, but since working at

HEM, she has frequented related meetings out of curiosity and because some patients and their relatives would ask about it. Accordingly, she did not participate out of "belief" or because she had to; she only wanted to respond to their questions and was open to any complementary approach that supports the well-being of patients, relatives, and staff members. She states:

> I perceive some differences from conventional therapy: some patients re-calibrate easier and faster with this spiritual aspect. [...] I do not know if I would call it a healing capacity; I personally believe so, but it is a very complex issue. I think these practices and related beliefs function as support complementary to other treatments, and I see a difference between patients who do and do not participate in Spiritist practices. They are more relaxed, serene, and calm, and if the person believes and internalizes this belief, there is a big chance that it will take you somewhere, and therapy will be more successful. They seem to cope better with their condition.
>
> (Interview 22 Feb. 2016)

Iotti refers to the dynamics of transforming meanings of experience toward explanatory models that enable patients to develop personal agency strategies with positive effects on their well-being. She laughs at my question if this might not be true for any religious or spiritual practice:

> I am already biased, but I believe Spiritism is more holistic. I developed an affinity for Spiritism because it provides answers other religions would not. It depends on the comprehensive level of a person; some patients are simple-minded, whereas Spiritism is very complex.
>
> (Interview 22 Feb. 2016)

It appears that Iotti, as a psychologist, mainly refers to the cognitive level of Spiritism in terms of how it might have the patients reflect on their experiences alongside with Kardec's doctrine and through the lectures or study groups they participate in, but she continues:

> There are patients over here whom I believe do not suffer from a psychiatric condition but are mediumistic – listening to voices, and so on. [...] I have at least to consider that this person is a medium, the same way I must consider biological dysfunction or the possibility of an inter-relatedness of both. [...] I usually check if my patients comply with pharmaceutical and psychotherapeutic treatments, but especially for patients affiliated with SUS, it is problematic as SUS only covers the costs of remedies but does not fund regular psychotherapy or continuous psychological attendance.
>
> (Interview 22 Feb. 2016)

Iotti considers that religious/spiritual engagement may complement conventional psychiatric treatment and fill a problematic economic and health-political gap. She further argues that, in some cases, conventional therapy might be a less promising approach than spiritual engagement:

We observe it: if a patient recovers after taking the remedies, we can be quite sure that it is a case of, let's say, acute schizophrenia. However, we can never be a hundred percent sure because we do not know how mediumship interacts with neurochemical processes. So, another approach would be to ask: what are the voices saying? We should explore implicit meanings, and if I feel that something "more" is involved, I sometimes suggest to patients to check on a Spiritist center. I am careful because they might not agree for religious or rational reasons, neglecting the existence of spirits or denying any interaction with them.
(Interview 22 Feb. 2016)

Even though Iotti does not identify as a Spiritist, she considers that there might be something beyond her formation as a psychologist and argues for healing cooperation as long as it serves the patients' well-being. She incorporates the spirit of complement so much that she devalues opposing positions as irrational and incomprehensible. She argues for a sober and unbiased evaluation of the diversity of cases and contexts:

My observation is that many internalized patients of HEM afterward start to frequent Spiritist centers. [...] Therefore, I believe that there should be even more integration of Spiritist practices, but we must be careful in terms of religious freedom and that we do not ideologically influence our patients. It is more about individually supporting the patients who are up for it. More study of Spiritism would help fight psychiatric patients' stigmatization.
(Interview 22 Feb. 2016)

Whereas Iotti explores the realm of Spiritist healing practices from a "rational" point of view in terms of more or less measurable experiences of therapy success and the general requirement of "professional open-mindedness" regarding divergent approaches to health, Osvaldo promotes a perspective that focuses on the affective implications of Spiritist engagement in (mental) healthcare. He is a medical doctor working at a public health center in Marília. He grew up in a Spiritist environment but detached from it until, three years ago, a dramatic family issue reconnected him with this practice that explains his experiences and related emotions. He declares that he was devastated after his wife divorced him, feeling sad, lost, and hateful at the same time, and he is convinced that what saved him was engaging at HEM. Now, for three months, he has co-organized the official transformation of HEM from a psychiatric hospital toward a polyclinic. To him, HEM differs from other psychiatric hospitals: it is "something more" that he perceives in the lectures and disobsession meetings, and that would help him to relax, recover, balance, and deal with his issues and experiences. He senses a strong connection between HEM and that "hospital on the spiritual plane," a "flow of energy" that affects him and could affect anybody:

> Besides supporting HEM as a volunteer, I see the necessity of cooperation because I worked in the health administration of Marilia. I know how many patients suffer from lack of treatment, and many more would suffer if HEM closed. Here, they are treated as humans and with love; they would hardly survive at home or in the street.
>
> (Interview 29 Jan. 2016)

Osvaldo connects several aspects that seem crucial for practices at HEM: healing cooperation between Spiritism, psychiatry, and biomedicine provides alternative explanatory models, charity as a practice of (self-)care, and sensory/affective levels. As chair of the Spiritist board, Vincente agrees with these aspects but appears to be more concerned with the distribution of sustained mental healthcare. He stresses the importance of HEM as an institution: the problem with the (de)institutionalization policy would be that public healthcare does not provide sufficient resources to maintain mental healthcare services, and thus, other resources would have to be sought. He supports the idea of patients being treated in their communities but complains that, in reality, psychiatric patients always have been, and under current circumstances will remain, marginal and abandoned. Especially within economically disadvantaged segments of society, families would have problems maintaining the care of their afflicted members. Regarding the purpose and effectiveness of Spiritist practices, he states:

> I think it is a good influence. What is *passe*? It is the renovation of your bioenergy and connection with spiritual levels. What does prayer do? You connect yourself to God independently from any religious denomination. You raise your thoughts to God, the creator. In the Bible, there are many passages about Jesus quarreling with God, his father, but then regulating himself by applying for His support. We must redirect to God, but the study is important, too: you can discuss the same work several times, but the interpretation will always be different. It opens our conscience, and this is what lectures are about. Even if the patients do not understand what the lecturer is talking about, the spirit listens, perceives, and receives important information. Moreover, the obsessing spirits also listen, which is the most important aspect of our work: they start to listen. We observe gradual changes in our patients, and I am sure they sometimes perceive more than it seems to us.
>
> (Interview 29 Jan. 2016)

I will further discuss the aspect of "listening" in Chapter 4, but Vincente's son Bruno also finds other words to explain HEM's spiritual tasks:

We do what we think is best for our patients, even if it means spiritually supporting them without their knowledge. [...] This is what love is about, and I believe that the professionals here are more than in other psychiatric hospitals trained to help, listen, and at least try to understand. There is more than daily routine: we try to add a more individual aspect of spiritual support, which greatly helps. [...] It helps the patients in a vibrational, energetic way. All these activities serve a culture of hope, solidarity, and interaction: nobody is alone; we are linked to each other. We create an environment of hope.

(Interview 03 Nov. 2015)

For several months, I frequented HEM regularly but rarely ever met one of the seven psychiatrists who would only see the patients for a few hours a day. Bruno and Vincente introduced me to Dr. Arlindo, who, for over 30 years, has worked as a psychiatrist at HEM. He performs one hour of group therapy several times a week and prescribes drugs. Being a psychiatrist, he postulates the preservation of psychiatric hospitals but wants to substitute long-term hospitalization with community-based treatment and complementary spiritual work. Being a Spiritist himself, he does not wish to proselytize anybody but believes that psychiatrists should engage with spiritual aspects or at least witness related procedures and integrate their observations into their medical records of patients. He declares:

The difference between HEM and other psychiatric hospitals is that we do not only work with spirituality but also offer spiritual formation. [...] Mental illness consists of many aspects, one being spiritual, and the spiritual aspect helps in therapy. I observed a positive effect of these practices in therapy. I would not argue that spirituality does the whole job, but it helps, sometimes not immediately, but at least supportive. [...] Lectures, evangelization, and *passe* are complementary forms of therapy, and it is not about the medium who miraculously heals but combining traditional psychotherapeutic treatment with Spiritist approaches to complement. [...] Even though it is a question of subjective perception, I see differences between patients who do or do not participate. I observe fewer back-laps and increasing ease and reflection. I cannot prove it, but I do see the difference. You might call these effects a form of healing, but I would be more careful and call it the support of a cure. [...] There could be, and there should be, more Kardecist treatment facilities as there is no doubt that they enhance our therapy success. It must be done, and it is not sufficient yet. It is a complementary technique to help people and deal with spirits simultaneously.

(Interview 19 Feb. 2016)

The example of Spiritist mental healthcare in Marília reveals a veritable dynamic of healing cooperation between health professionals, spirits, mediums, and clients/patients, constituting a space of medical and spiritual complement. Various institutions form a network on a local, national, international (see Chapter 5), and even "transdimensional" level (as with the hospital in the spiritual sphere), providing spiritual progress through lectures, study groups, mediumship practices, fraternal care, and energetic treatments. It connects human healers and patients with entities such as God, Jesus, and spirits, but also with other actants and agencies such as books, water, and energies/fluids, all linked with the voices of lecturers, mediums, and voluntary caretakers. Here, I want to focus on the triangular interaction of discarnate spirits (afflicting and healing ones), patients/clients, and healers (biomedical and psychiatric therapists, mediums, and Spiritist volunteers). As the case studies, observations, and interview excerpts illustrate, some patients/clients and volunteers/mediums of HEM and CELV have been through troubling experiences and would hardly or not at all feel relief by sole biomedical, psychiatric, or religious treatments. Within the framework of Spiritist healing practices, they can communicate their problems to somebody who listens to them for as long as necessary. The volunteers ask questions, calm down the afflicted, and direct the conversation toward the persons' responsibility, agency, and self-healing capacities without blaming them or others. This form of guided spiritual development and the discussion of possible causes of affliction implicates the need for the patients to actively work on their behavior and regularly participate in subsequent practices such as lectures, evangelization sessions, and energetic treatment. Many continue frequenting the centers, attending study groups and mediumship training sessions, and months or years later become volunteers themselves. The declared purpose is to facilitate personal progress toward self-responsibility, (self-)care, and agency in coping with (illness) experiences. Moreover, these practices distribute explanatory models substituting psychiatric discourse on external (social) and internal (organic) causes of affliction with perspectives on external and internal spiritual factors.

Where Theissen (2009) observes practices of guilt and moral control (see Chapter 2), I suggest that Spiritist explanatory models produce a frame to negotiate internal and external factors of affliction and healing, avoiding stigmatization, social exclusion, and experiences of patiency. The case studies reveal a dynamic of how explanatory models within Kardecist mental healthcare address the self-responsibility of patients to a certain degree. Far from stigmatizing the experience of affliction, they offer consolation, meaning, and coping strategies. Accordingly, they facilitate strategies of active (agency) instead of passive (patiency) coping (cf. Lott 2016). Regina's and Elisângela's cases serve as examples of this opposition. From the perspective of psychiatric diagnostic standards (e.g., ICD-10; cf. WHO 2016), both develop a disposition for an affective disorder with extraordinary sensory perceptions (hallucinations) in context with the loss of beloved ones: Regina "listens" to voices; Elisângela "sees things" and feels "cursed and harassed" by spiritual entities. Both are of comparable social backgrounds (urban middle class, teachers) and must cope with unexpected life situations. Still, Regina never becomes a psychiatric patient. Her experience is interpreted as mediumship and the influence of obsessing spirits (in this case, benevolent ones). She experiences how, in the Kardecist context, people make sense of her story in spiritual terms and support her in resolving her issues. She starts to study Kardecist doctrine and integrates related discourse and practice into her daily habits, supporting and consoling others who suffer from comparable afflictions. She actively works on and with her experience in a community that does not stigmatize but appreciates it. Comparing it with the other narratives regarding a processional engagement with Spiritism, it seems a typical pattern for people participating in Kardecist practice: few were raised as Spiritists or, like William, turned to it out of curiosity. Most had disturbing experiences and found relief within the Spiritist centers. They do not necessarily develop mediumship but find explanations for their health problems, bad luck, social experiences, or conflicts, and start to work on themselves not because they feel guilty for what happened to them but because they feel responsible for changing their fortune.

Elisângela has not been as lucky: she twice became a psychiatric patient of HEM but now tends to develop a similar coping strategy. She feels guilty for the death of her friends and has been treated as "mad" by her peers as soon as she communicated her experiences to them. Being able to discuss concepts of mediumship and obsession provides her with an explanation and the possibility to develop agency. She already applied these concepts in the past but used them as an excuse for her condition; now, she perceives it as a gift to share with others. Elisângela takes it as her obligation to support others in their spiritual progress, and already throughout her hospitalization at HEM, she feels responsible for other patients and the *gringo* anthropologist, wanting to share all her knowledge, love, and affection. Her plans for the future imply that she will contribute to Kardecist practices in her hometown, just like Regina and William would do here. It seems to be a regular pattern of healing and engagement that I observe with many patients/clients of HEM and CELV. For example, like Ana-Paula, many patients of HEM start to frequent Spiritist centers after being released from psychiatric treatment, especially after suffering from relapses. Others, like Regina, Osvaldo, and (hopefully) Janina and Sabrina, do not become patients but likewise experience consolation and develop coping strategies by permanently engaging with Spiritism. To sum up, all my interlocutors share the conviction that at least some factors of Spiritist healing practices would support their current well-being: (1) the experience of the *passe*, the enlightenment through the lectures, and the personal development by study and charity, (2) a particular frame and structure providing social backup and the feeling of doing something useful, and (3) the fact that dealing with spiritual issues seems to be more socially accepted than "madness." Many start to engage as volunteers to not only take care of themselves but also for others, trying to find answers to their life questions, developing strategies to cope with their problems and afflictions, and experiencing consolation by "sharing and caring."

Thiesbonenkamp-Maag (2014), in her investigation of spiritual healing and caring practices of Philippine migrants in Germany, elaborates how self-care and care are interconnected in karmic, moral, and/or ethical terms: to help others also improves the (spiritual) condition of the supporter, and therefore, activates self-healing capacities for both. Caring for others implies self-care in terms of sharing experiences, but also supporting others with personal experiences and thus providing and gaining social and spiritual support. Thiesbonenkamp-Maag defines care as a "technology of the self" (ibid.: 136ff; cf. Foucault 1988b) but also integrates aspects of "social capital" and "agency" (cf. Bourdieu 1977; Giddens 1979) into her model of (self-)care. This perspective implies not to view humans as individual entities but as relational beings dependent on and shaped by interaction. Translated to the Spiritist context, lectures, evangelization sessions, and fraternal care aim at simultaneously developing self-responsibility, (self-)love, and charity as interconnected practices. Especially at HEM, I observed a strong solidarity among the patients and various forms of reciprocal care. Therapeutic progress and success, from this perspective, do not solely depend on medicalization or individual models of psycho- and occupational therapy but on a process and dynamic of interaction that connects "Selves" and "Others" in an enactment of empathy and mutual support (cf. Thiesbonenkamp-Maag 2014: 125f; see Chapter 4). Within mediumship and disobsession practices, the "Other" is extended to the spiritual sphere, and related practices of communication, interaction, and mutual support connect the spiritual and material worlds. Waldram (2013), in this regard, distinguishes healing practices that address the restoration ("cure") of the well-being of a person from those promoting personal transformation ("heal") as a coping strategy where the patient is not restored to a former state but guided toward a new habitus and perception of self, others, illness, and health. I interpret Kardecist healing practices as such a transformational approach.

The vignettes and case studies reveal a variety of healing cooperation models that integrate Spiritist explanatory models and healing practices into conventional mental healthcare. HEM and CELV constitute examples of symmetrical and almost symbiotic healing cooperation between Spiritists and psychiatrists. The administration of HEM organizes the cooperation between biomedically educated psychiatrists, other health professionals, and voluntary, religiously oriented individuals associated with the various Spiritist centers of Marília. The case studies of Ana-Paula and Elisângela demonstrate how healing cooperation is shaped by a complement of "medicalization" and "evangelization," resulting in gradual recovery with progressive spiritual engagement. There is more to Spiritist healing practices than being a substitute or a complement to biomedical or psychiatric treatment. It is about the relationship between Self and Others.

Notes

1   Three weeks before, on 05 November 2015, a basin of mining leftovers busted in Mariana (Minas Gerais/Brazil), leaving a whole region covered in poisonous mud and killing a contested number of people.
2   The spirit's gender is not identified, but the way William addresses it, I imagine the male sex.
3   Interestingly, this 8-week treatment reminds me of comparable timeframes in mindfulness training adapted to psychotherapy (see Kabat-Zinn 2003). I will return to the parallels in Chapter 4.
4   I was asked not to share it, so I will not display it here.

Aesthetics of Healing

A Sense of Self and Other

On a Thursday night in November 2015, hundreds of visitors flock to the Spiritist center CELV, where mediums supposedly will communicate messages from the deceased through psychography. Infinite rows of white plastic chairs are arranged in front of a stage with a large table and wooden chairs. A screen next to the stage flashes images of beautiful landscapes, and speakers purr a decelerated and meditative instrumental version of Louis Armstrong's "What a Wonderful World." Then, geese flocks and panda families appear on the screen while prayers to God, Jesus, and benevolent spirits echo from the speakers, pledging their support. CELV's administrator, César, picks up the microphone at precisely 8:00 p.m. and welcomes everyone to this special occasion. He declares that not all will be able to receive messages from beloved ones but that witnessing life after death and the possibility of communication should console all mourners and provide hope to the desperate. Besides the aesthetic effects of the introductory music and screening, it is his voice that affects me: his speech manifests into a one-hour sermon on reincarnation, karma, spiritual progress, and self-responsibility, and the monotonic melody of his voice develops a hypnotizing effect. Unlike other Brazilian religious environments I have witnessed, he does not yell, scream, or intone chants, and participants do not disrupt the sermon – no one whispers or comments to their neighbor; no restless movements or kids running around, just silence, concentration, and devotion.

Afterward, an older man reads a few paragraphs from "The Gospel According to Spiritism" (Kardec 2008) and speaks the Lord's Prayer. At 9:30 p.m., six mediums sit down around the table, close their eyes, and seem to concentrate on what appears to be some inner perception. They write down messages on little sheets of paper that assistants then read out loud. Some are quite detailed, mentioning names, situations, and intimate information, provoking sobbing and sighs in the audience. Others are quite unspecific and might apply to anyone's expectations. Later, I will learn that the quality of mediumistic messages depends on the medium's spiritual progress and acquired skills. I, therefore, have wondered how mediumship skills are learned, elaborated, and scaled. I have become interested in what

DOI: 10.4324/9781032637167-4

happens to participants of mediumship practices on the experiential level, and this curiosity dragged me into the realm of mediumship practices as a core element of Spiritist mental healthcare in Brazil. The vignette reminds us again of the centrality of reading, lecturing, listening, and involved sensory aspects. Asking Cesar and other lecturers afterward, they state that they often even prepare some elements for the introduction but would then speak intuitively (Session 26 Nov. 2015).

Chapter 2 highlighted the historical entanglement of Spiritism and psychiatry, emphasizing the Brazilian mental healthcare system and introducing the concepts of "obsession" and "mediumship." In a further step, Chapter 3 displayed my observations of Spiritist mental healthcare practices as healing cooperation between Spiritists and psychiatrists, integrating the narratives of involved individuals (patients, mediums, therapists, Spiritist volunteers, and myself as a participant observer). I have already mentioned the performative character of practices and that they produce embodied and sensory relief in participants. In this chapter, I intend to further develop this approach by linking my ethnographic accounts to a theoretical framework that investigates experiential, embodied, and sensory therapeutic aspects. It focuses on the embodiment of spirits and also presents some autoethnographic accounts of my experiences in mediumship practices. As Edith Turner (2010: 218) puts it, spirits are experiences, and their ethnography is a transformative experience on its own. Accordingly, by exploring my perceptions and personal experiences as a participant observer – or, as it will turn out to be, an observing participant – I intend to analyze aesthetic aspects of healing to explore what in reminiscence to Csordas (1994) we may call a phenomenology of a "spiritual self." This chapter addresses the delimitations and dissolutions of Self and Other as interconnected agencies, unsettling Cartesian-derived dualistic notions of Body–Mind, Human–Spirit, Self–Other, Patient–Healer, or Participant–Observer. Any given social situation might serve a specific functionality and respond to external structures, but it is developed by – and creates – interconnected agencies. This insight raises the question of how far agencies within the frame of mental healthcare interrelate as Self and Other and if this delimitation of categories might not be fluid, contextual, and negotiable (cf. Desjaralais & Throop 2011: 91). I will, therefore, explore how various agencies shape healing experiences and create effectiveness on a sensory, embodied, and interactional level.

Throughout the previous chapters, I have discussed observations and experiences of Spiritist healing practices, aligned them to the narratives of my interlocutors, and developed a preliminary conclusion that implies the interpretation of Spiritist mental healthcare practices as healing cooperation of various institutions and actors. They contribute to a sustained experience of health, well-being, and coping, especially regarding social participation and integration factors: self-care and care for others are interconnected.

Conceptualizations, definitions, and the relatedness of categories like Selves and Others thus appear crucial when exploring Spiritist mental healthcare. In this regard, Kirmayer (1989a) argues that psychotherapeutic interventions depend on the social formation of the patients. He describes how in "Western psychotherapy," (1) the self applies to a concept of the human as an autonomous, individual being, and (2) narrative practices and the cognitive discussion of emotional states address afflictions of the self. He juxtaposes this model to the perspective of dividual selves who would not identify with individual autonomy but their interrelatedness with others, including non-human beings (e.g., totems, spirits, ancestors, animals, plants, and objects). Just like in the paradigmatic discussion by Nichter (1981) on the idioms of distress among Brahman women in India, verbally articulated complaints on inner emotional states and experiences appear pointless because problems are not located in the person, self, or individual body but in the realm of relationships and interaction. Therapists, therefore, would have to explore these realms and related coping strategies, and Kirmayer (1989b), in this regard, identifies the concept of "mind" as one of the most challenging categories regarding the negotiation of "Western" and "non-Western" approaches to Self, questioning the (universal) validity of Cartesian dualism as a concept of the self/person that defines mind as an agency distinct from bodily perceptions.

Eller (2019) develops a more distinguished perspective on individual–dividual differentiation, exploring how various societies, and even different members of a social group, do not simply apply to one of these strict categories but oscillate between intersubjectivity and egocentrism as loci of Self (ibid.: 126f). Different categories of personhood would affect the spheres of mental health and healthcare as they constitute local ethno-psychologies (ibid.: 118). Moreover, they are often framed by discursive and bodily techniques (or technologies of self, cf. Bourdieu 1977; Mauss 1985; Foucault 1988b), and Eller (2019: 118f) elaborates how concepts of self or personhood usually imply the adaption to a distinctive socially sanctioned *habitus* and moral value system, stressing that also non-human agencies are of relevance (ibid.: 134f). This is also the case for Spiritism in Brazil: the notion of the person consists of a tripartite model including the body, the *perispirit*, and the spirit. Whereas the body serves as a material container of lived experience, the *perispirit* implies spiritual/karmic elements to be resolved, and a person's Self is located in the spirit, which develops throughout many lifetimes. Accordingly, and comparing different cultural models on the self and the person worldwide, Eller (ibid.: 122f) describes a person's constitution as "self-work" in terms of integration and transformation of bodily, mental, and spiritual elements. It implies bodily, affective, and sensory experiences, and this is the experiential sphere I refer to as the Aesthetics of Healing in the context of Spiritist mental healthcare.

I will discuss ritualized techniques as sensory manipulation of perception beyond symbolical, metaphorical, or imaginary frames of meaning; they affect participants on a sensory level and contribute to an experience of healing. Accordingly, I will investigate practices of stimuli reduction and enhancement and explore the realm of "voices" as central sensory triggers in the interaction of patients, healers, and spirits and in the production of a sixth sense that, emically, is referred to as mediumship. Furthermore, whereas many anthropological studies on mediumship healing focus on the role of the "medium as a self-healed healer," I will elaborate on how sensory-perceptual manipulations affect all participants and aim at the transformation of their self-perception, habits, and interaction with others. It implies investigating how explanatory models and related practices help to reframe experiences from being interpreted as deviant, anti-social behavior toward a "natural" spiritual phenomenon to be integrated into social practice.

Performance and Embodiment of Healing

I have listened to a common idiom for years and witnessed it reproducing within different social settings: "sharing is caring." In Chapter 3, I discussed how care and self-care intersect in spiritual terms. Here, I want to take it further: sharing involves reciprocal bodily practices, including, e.g., studying together, lecturing, providing fraternal care, and *passe*, in short, interacting. The core aspect of my conceptualization of the Aesthetics of Healing transgresses the performative use of symbols and other audio–visual stimuli and elaborates on the sensory engagement of people who interact, communicate, cope with their conditions, and develop strategies for counteracting them. Several researchers have investigated Brazilian Spiritist practices as performative enactments of social conflict, metacommunication on experienced live worlds and social challenges, or as psycho-social strategies to integrate afflicted individuals into a peer group of fellows. Unfortunately, many of these studies do not reflect on, or at least consider, emic notions of Self as divergent from the researchers' etic bias. They apply "Western" psychological and explanatory models to serve their interpretation of observed practices but lack insight into how their interlocutors experience, perceive, and sense therapeutic interventions. To my knowledge, only Greenfield (2008) at least considers "biological-cultural" aspects of Spiritist healing practices and discusses related sensory/affective elements. However, instead of systematically exploring them, he produces a reductionist narrative on the "bodyliness of Brazilians" and assumes a general openness to altered states of consciousness that facilitate perceptional manipulation by "hypnosis and suggestion." I agree with Rocha (2017), who stresses that this line of argument invokes cultural preassumptions and prejudice rather than providing any insight on *how* and *why* exactly Spiritist healing practices are of such disproportionate importance for the Brazilian healthcare sector when compared to, for example, the USA or Europe (see Chapters 2 and 5). However, in earlier studies, Greenfield (1992, 2004) mentions performative aspects of disobsession as enactments of "social drama" and "morality play." His observation regards practices where patients/clients participate in mediumistic sessions and witness the evangelization of "their obsessors." However, throughout my investigation of Kardecist healing practices in Marília and beyond, I hardly ever noticed something comparable. On the contrary, disobsession and mediumship sessions usually explicitly exclude patients or clients due to legal implications and avoid the exteriorization of responsibilities by patients. Nonetheless, the performative lens might be of some analytical value regarding the actual participants of mediumship sessions and their experiences when considering that many engage in those care practices by means of self-care.

From an anthropological perspective, I assume that any healing practice is a "rite of passage" that transforms participants, particularly patients, who are guided from a state of affliction toward an experience of well-being. I will still return to the question of how Spiritist healing practices generally apply to this notion, but at this level of analytical argument, I want to focus on "healers" who have been "patients" or could have become so if not for their engagement with Spiritist practice. It is another well-known concept among both healers and medical anthropologists that usually, in many cultures, the "decision" to become a spirit medium, a healer, or a shaman is an involuntary process and imposes narratives of the "wounded healer" who transforms traumatic experiences toward a coping strategy by supporting others. In reminiscence, but also as inversion, of Goethe's Sorcerer's Applicant (*Zauberlehrling*), it appears that participants of disobsession summon the spirits they cannot dispose of. It provides ritual structures with sequences of separation (meeting in a small group, closing the doors, reducing any external stimuli), liminality (initiated by lectures and prayers), and re-entry (final prayers and returning home), producing a sense of communitas in terms of solidary engagement against spiritual obsessors. Simultaneously, participants perform an antistructure in that it is not the spirits who afflict the humans but that the latter instruct the former in terms of stopping their menace and, in an act of love and charity, guiding them toward an experience of healing on another spiritual level. It is a "gentle exorcism" that does not condemn but helps the simultaneously afflicted and afflicting spirits (see Chapter 3). At the same time, it is a "morality play" as many spirits display behaviors that most participants do not approve of, e.g., substance abuse, promiscuity, or violence. Habits of charity, love, and care are enacted to overcome these menaces and to serve as an ideal scheme for everyday life.

From this perspective, the healers are the healed as they develop coping strategies within their lifeworld that they share with others. The performance helps them to overcome their doubts parallel to the indoctrination of the spirits following its structured pattern: the obsessing spirits contradict Spiritist knowledge, but their human counterparts instruct them on how to apply it. When the spirits surrender, they experience joy and "healing," consolidating knowledge and habit for all participants who witness this process. As Regina puts it: "It proves that this is real" (Interview 07 Jan. 2016). The performance, therefore, includes metacommunication on experienced realities on various levels: many social conflicts are displayed in the spirit's narratives, and it seems that they engage against selfish practices in an unequal society. At the same time, Spiritists justify these inequalities with the spiritual progress of humans and the lessons they must learn. They criticize an alleged pronounced and immanent materiality, corporeality, and lustfulness within Brazilian culture and preach self-discipline and spiritual engagement. They thus produce an antistructure to a perceived reality and attempt to display veritable communitas in the sense of social equality, mutual care, and rational, respectful behavior. In this, they also criticize the official healthcare system, where these qualities are seemingly lacking. In this regard, aspects of hospital mimicry in Spiritist healing practices (cf. Maués 2003) play a double role: within disobsession, the imagination of a hospital on the spiritual plane displays an ideal of healthcare that Brazilian health policy does not provide (see Chapters 2 and 3).

Apart from this example, HEM and CELV provide other instances of hospital mimicry, e.g., the image of *passe* as an "energetic transfusion," the consumption of "fluidized" water as a remedy, the fraternal attendance as an anamnesis and psychological consultation, and the evangelization as psychotherapeutic group therapy. In other Spiritist centers (see Chapter 5; cf. Greenfield 2008; Rocha 2017), alleged spirit doctors incorporate in a medium and supported by a staff of nurses and health assistants, energetically treat patients in a hospital-like environment with waiting rooms where instead of the newspaper or gossip magazine, people read Spiritist literature, and treatment rooms consist of stretchers and clinical furniture, shelves of patient's files, liquids in bottles, band-aids, etc. As I will further explore in Chapter 5, these institutions often do not serve as a complement to biomedicine or psychiatry but as alternatives or even substitutes for marginal official healthcare resources. Staff members, mediums, and even incorporated spirit doctors admitted that they chose to work in such an aesthetic environment because patients would believe more in therapy success when they sensorily experience a space that cognitively reminds them of a clinic. The performance would enhance their coping behavior.

For the cases of HEM and CELV, we might even assume an "academia mimicry" once the practices of lectures and study groups appear reasonably elaborate and structured, displaying alleged rational scientific approaches and procedures. I do not interpret it as a symbolic pretension but as a veritable Third Space (cf. Bhabha 1994) of hybridizing scientific, medical, psychiatric, religious, and spiritual knowledge and practice that aims at transforming and reframing experience. By communicating explanatory models of mediumship, obsession, and the urge for spiritual progress within the various Spiritist healing practices, "abnormal" experiences and behavior are reinterpreted from a psychiatric problem to a spiritual one. By discussing and performing spiritual issues as a common trait everybody is involved in resolving, Spiritism thus applies a sense of "normality" and acknowledges patients' agency. They discard habits of victimization and avoid stigmatization as spiritual engagement in Brazil is socially more accepted, esteemed, and integrative than a psychiatric diagnosis, which, in opposition to diverse political efforts, still includes social marginalization or exclusion (see Chapter 2). Rödiger (2003: 32f), with a focus on the habitualization of the "Brazilian body," describes such processes as a negotiation of inner selves with their social environments, simultaneously structuring and being structured by cognition, norms, aesthetic values, practice, and interaction in a somewhat compulsory fashion.

Several vignettes in Chapter 3 illustrate how Spiritists gradually transform from afflicted individuals toward (self-)caring beings by incorporating a "Spiritist habitus." It appears to be a rather cognitive process considering the importance of lectures and study groups, but I argue that bodily/sensory aspects do play a significant role here, let alone the practice of *passe*: it is not just a form of bodily attention or interaction but a practice that serves the reflection and incorporation of previously listened lectures in total silence and self-focus. Terencio shared his interpretation of *passe* with me, describing it as a "transfusion of energies," which, in a way, displays the aforementioned aspects of hospital mimicry. However, he also explained it to me as a technique to manipulate self-perception and sensory experience: it serves to internalize certain values and explore and sensitize inner worlds and experiences. However, although neuro-anthropological approaches regard ritualization and repetition of practices as affecting experiences due to endocrine and neuronal processes, I remain critical of how bodily and cultural aspects complement each other here. It does not appear sufficient to argue that certain spiritual practices trigger some form of bodily perception or experience. Therefore, I suggest that we must dig deeper and explore what happens at the sensory level as an interface of individual, social, and religious-spiritual-philosophical levels of perception, experience, belief, and knowledge.

Various studies on Brazilian Spiritism (cf. Schmidt 2016a; Rocha 2017) and other healing practices that engage with spirits, such as Cuban *Espiritismo* (cf. Espirito Santo 2015), Afro-Brazilian religions (cf. Seligman 2014; Pierini 2020), or Pentecostalism (cf. Rabelo et al. 2009) usually stress the importance of "embodied learning" in terms of cultivating a new form of (self-)perception. They conceptualize the self as a permanent project of a continuous learning process to deal with particular emotional states and as a training to shift attention from cognitive perception toward internal factors and bodily processes. Schmidt (2016a: 150), therefore, stresses the aspect of mediumship as a practice to develop agency and resolve personal issues within a given social environment. Accordingly, Seligman (2005), for the example of mediumship experiences in Afro-Brazilian *Candomblé*, argues that

> [A]ltered states of consciousness should not be considered the central and defining element of mediumship. An alternative model is proposed, in which the combination of social conditions and somatic susceptibilities causes certain individuals to identify with the mediumship role [...]. [D]issociation is not a pathological experience, but [...] a therapeutic mechanism, learned through religious participation.
>
> (Seligman 2005: 71)

Seligman addresses an important issue: mediumship as a practice offers explanatory models to reframe experiences, strategies to cope with them, and a therapeutic effect related to religious engagement (ibid.). She elaborates on her argument that related healing practices aim to deconstruct, repair, and incorporate a sense of Self through bodily mechanisms and experiences (ibid. 2010: 297). She interprets mediumship as a cultural tool to contribute to the transformation of cognitive and bodily experiences of incoherence to facilitate processes of recoherence by bodily engagement and involved forms of self-healing. Seligman (2014: 159f) concludes that ritual spirit possession links inner (self-)perception to outer role expectations and, as an enactment, displays transformations of subjectivity and selfhood in terms of self-healing and (re)adjustment of internal and external senses of Self. At first sight, bodily and sensory engagement does not seem to play a significant role in Kardecist practices, but I suggest further exploring related sensory environments and investigating how they impact health, illness, and healing.

Mediumship Experiences

Asking Vincente about the importance of disobsession practices for HEM and its' patients, he answers:

> It is, first, about mediumship. Many people do not know that they have this capacity and get diagnosed with schizophrenia or something like that. However, sometimes, it is mediumship, and people do not know how to use this gift. These sessions are important for the hospital to provide clarity for both sides: for the incarnate and the discarnate.
>
> (Interview 01 Dec. 2015)

Accordingly, a significant aspect of disobsession is to gain and share spiritual knowledge with the help of mediums. It does not exclusively rely on auditive communication; psychographic messages are also received and then read aloud. Within Vincente's disobsession group that William guides (see Chapter 3), Wilson would do so in a session one month after I arrived in Marília: "With the blessing of Jesus, distraction, laziness, and adversity disappear right away" (Session 01 Dec. 2015), a formula that from now on, he would repeat in every meeting and have other participants also repeating it in a mantra type style. On the same occasion, he passes to me a piece of paper with an alleged personal psychographic message: *Helmar, vence-se pela continuidade, pela persistência, pelo coragem de todas as dias como a água vence a pedra.* ("Helmar, overcome yourself by continuity, persistence, and courage every single day the same way the water polishes the stone."). I mention it here because I perceive it as relating to comments on my person the previous week when I had strange sensory perceptions throughout a disobsession meeting that so far I have not commented on but that later, upon my communication, several Spiritists would refer to as a mediumship ability: right after the Lord's Prayer, I started to shiver and shake and would feel a pain in my chest just before a spirit would through a medium complain about his death experience of a heart attack. Shortly after, I would feel angry and aggressive, wanting to throw chairs and tables. Right after, an outraged and aggressive spirit incorporated into a medium and aggressively complained about his situation. It makes me wonder how far this capacity of "mediumship" relates to qualities of empathy, intuition, and/or sensory interaction. How could he "know" about my experiences, doubts, and resistance? I could never ask him because, even though he invited me to several meetings and sessions, we never had a private conversation or interview. Instead, I asked Vincente to clarify my confusion:

> Yes, we feel it! We get a good impression of what is going on over there, of how the spiritual team works. [...] It is intuitive, and many of us get the whole thing already, even before the spirit talks. [...] I do not even know if this is intuition or already mediumship or if intuition is mediumship. Sometimes, we feel the spirits pass by, giving us a heavy feeling, and then the spiritual guides come and alleviate us. You stay happy, and then suddenly, you stay sad. We dedicate this one hour a week to the discarnate spirits surrounding us. Some of them are hateful, and they tear you down; others are helpful and lift you. When they come, you feel it right away. You feel it physically because the aura and the fluids affect you. It is the contact of aura with aura, which makes you feel what you feel. Sometimes, this feeling is unspecific, but sometimes it is something you feel on your arm, in your belly, or thoughts that are not yours. You have different thoughts. It is their thoughts, and you are receiving them. [...] After a reunion, I feel better; the heavy sensations disappear. The session itself is full of issues and troubles to be resolved, for them to resolve, but I leave more at ease, calm ... more normal.
>
> (Interview 01 Dec. 2015)

I take it as a hint of how participants intensely engage with these practices on an affective/sensory level and how they also concern themselves. However, it would not stop there; another formative experience occurred on a Friday morning in January 2016: Spiritist volunteers and administration members of HEM gather for a mediumistic session to receive messages from "spiritual mentors" as guidelines for their practice. The course and structure of the meeting do not differ much from other mediumship sessions (see Chapter 3), only that participants seem to be more relaxed, and the spirits' communications through mediums appear to be calmer. Even though the windows are closed with curtains, and the light is dimmed, the room seems to shine bright. The session starts with a lecture on love, charity, and the importance of prayer-as-energy before absolute silence captures the space for several minutes. Usually, throughout these intervals, I would hear cars, motorbikes, barking dogs, or some distorted pitch of a nearby television, but today, there are only birdsongs and some screeching parrots passing by. It is a feeling of total peace and harmony, and I almost fall asleep. When, finally, the medium Bruno starts to communicate a spiritual message, he is interrupted by knocking at the door, and a delivery boy brings cake for the group to have with coffee after the session. Nobody seems to be irritated, but I experience it as a disruption. The lad leaves and closes the door, but twice, it opens again for no evident reason. Being already so intimate with Spiritist perspectives, I wonder if some disturbing spirits are mocking us. However, when Osvaldo finally manages to close the door, someone else gets up to look for the coffee that should have come with the cake. William arrives twenty minutes late, and I stay confused: throughout my research in Marília, I have been told how essential skills of discipline and punctuality would be as the spirits also have their obligations and appointments. I understand that many Brazilians have a different idea of discipline and punctuality than I do as the son of a German soldier. However, I feel so distorted and torn out of my comfort zone that I develop negative, if not aggressive, feelings about the situation. I now really believe that an evil spirit is haunting the place and simultaneously begin to question my sanity. Afterward, some participants agree that they had similar experiences, but they would not talk about it to not give power to it. I do not remember in detail the subsequent mediumistic messages because even my voice recorder has refused to work and only produces distorted fragments of this incident. I recall that I start to think of a good friend who has suffered from incurable cancer and will die a few days later. I am crying and silently begin to pray for the first time in ages. Then, a medium transmits a message of the co-founder and now spiritual mentor of HEM Manoel Saad, communicating images of light and positive energy. The whole room suddenly appears to shine with bright golden sunbeams even though the curtains are closed. My sadness transforms into something joyful, and in front of "my inner eye," I "see" what I can best describe as pulsating and transforming energy fields: first blue and green, then subsequently they

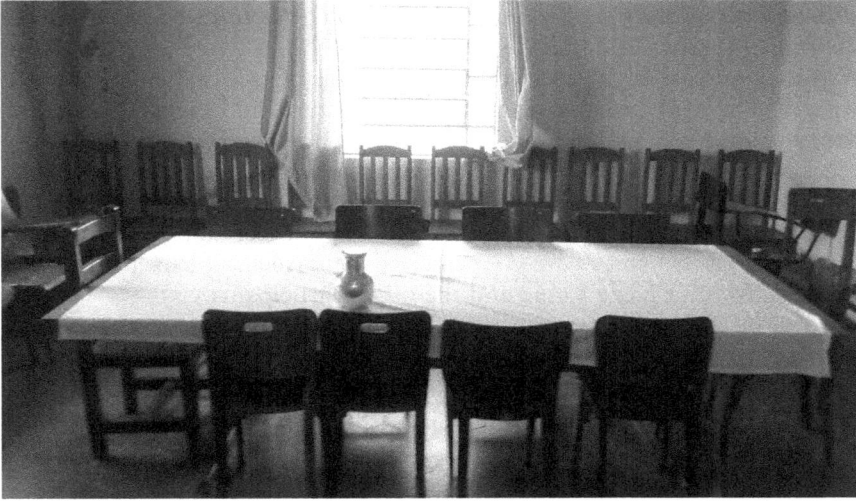

Figure 4.1 HEM's *Sala Mediúnica* (Mediumship Room) (Photography by HK 2015).

become violet, red, orange, yellow, and finally bright white. I realize human-shaped shadows passing by, and twice, I even see "faces" coming close to me. I cannot describe their features, but I feel their gaze. It is a very soothing and comfortable experience. I recall that years ago, I had a similar experience in an *Umbanda* ceremony but ascribed it to trance-induced imagination after sleepless hours of dance, ritual engagement, and a certain knowledge of what I was expected to see and feel. Today, it seems to be different: nobody told me what would happen or in any other way would shape my imagination to produce an experience which, independent from each other, other participants afterward narrate that they shared: the room is shining white and golden, and everybody experiences it as a blessing. As I cannot ascribe my perceptions to imagination based on other persons' accounts, I am convinced that now, after several months of participation in various mediumistic groups, I have increasingly attuned to these practices triggering a certain kind of "inner" sensory perception, so much that I even comprehend "things" similar to fellow participants' perceptions (Session 29 Jan. 2016) (Figure 4.1).

It has not been my first, nor will it be my last mesmerizing experience. Regina has introduced me to her friend Maria-Helena, who takes care of people with similar experiences within specific mediumship training courses. There, they learn how to control and use them for the sake of others (both incarnate and discarnate spirits). I meet her at her home, and she declares that in the 37 years she has lived in Marília – half of her life – she explored 13 different religious denominations before ending up with Spiritism about 20 years ago. Apart from all her other religious-spiritual experiments,

Kardecism would be the only one to convince her due to its emphasis on the importance of study and knowledge. For years, she has worked as a nurse in HEM and increasingly witnessed the importance of spiritual engagement in therapy. However, she criticizes the focus on lectures and evangelization and instead proposes to explore and train patients' mediumship skills. She also argues for integrating concepts of *chakras* and energetic fields as they would transform the reception of *passe* as a treatment on a different level (see Chapter 5). She explains that my recent experiences apply to this idea because she is convinced that I perceived benevolent spirits providing a particular form of *passe* to me and the other participants.

Maria-Helena argues that treating any affliction should consist of spiritual and material approaches to address the spirit, the *perispirit*, and the body. Only this triangular combination would holistically address the issues of a person, and once she perceives humans as holistic beings, medicine would have to become a holistic science integrating these aspects. She reports that she became a Spiritist while working at HEM because she witnessed so many impacts on patients that she could only understand in mediumship terms. However, according to her, mediumship training at HEM and CELV is a recent development and still does not integrate psychiatric patients as there have been many conflicts over the question of whether they should not be morally guided instead of using mediumship as an "excuse" (Interview 18 Feb. 2016). Taylor, a board member of CELV's administration, defines mediumship as a sensory and mental connection where humans and spirits syntonize. The medium becomes an intermediator to facilitate communication. He declares that every human being is a medium but that it depends on the bodily constitution and composition and how elaborate the capacity is. There are different types of mediumship (e.g., seeing, hearing, and intuition), and all mediums have unique ways of connecting and perceiving through their *perispirit*. He suggests I participate in a mediumship study and training group to explore this human property of care, well-being, and progress (Interview 22 Nov. 2015).

Those who become mediums complete veritable training in various study groups. To be accepted as a participant in regular mediumship and disobsession meetings, a person has to study Kardecist literature for at least three years before completing several training courses. One of these courses is directed by Magali, the wife of William. It displays a pattern similar to "regular" mediumship sessions, except that more time is spent reading Spiritist literature and discussing mediumistic experiences. I participated in a session in January 2016 that lasted about 2 hours and comprised 15 persons, mainly women between 25 and 45 years old. At the beginning of the session, everybody in the room concentrates in silence while a mix of classical and New Age music plays in the background. For the next 45 minutes, different participants read various Spiritist texts aloud. Magali chimes in tranquility, contributing comments, reflections, and discussions on the mentioned topics.

Finally, she asks somebody to intuitively speak a prayer to God, Jesus, and the benevolent spirits. Simultaneously, the doors and windows are closed, and the light is extinguished. Another person recites the Lord's Prayer, while others silently provide *passe* to everybody. Spiritual communication starts immediately: different voices overlap, and following what is said in particular situations is hard. I observe Magali, who is now going around from person to person. She asks if everything is alright and instructs them to "let it out." Magali provides *passe* to a young woman covered in tears and tells her that this sadness is not hers and that she must speak the Lord's Prayer to recover. In between, I hear screams such as, "My daughter, I have to return!" or "Help!" I feel pain in my left shoulder, arm, and around my chest for some time, as I have a vision of a man falling to the floor, suffering from a heart attack, and crying for help. Not knowing what to do, I also pray until I feel relief. Strong emotions are channeled, and many feel sickness or pain. Magali continues to walk around, asking if everybody is alright, and if not, telling them to pray the Lord's Prayer. Several of these "rounds" occur, the most disturbing being a simultaneous experience by several participants witnessing the slaughtering of pregnant women and their unborn children somewhere in Africa. Many start weeping and crying out; it is tough to bear. It takes a while before participants become observably exhausted and finally return to silence. A prayer expressing the desire to cleanse participants of these experiences concludes the session. The door is opened, the light is switched on, and everyone drinks a cup of water and departs. Some people stay and talk in groups or wait for a quick exchange with Magali. I leave immediately, feeling overwhelmed with contradictory emotions (Session 23 Jan. 2016).

In an interview a week later, Magali also expresses her conviction that I am a medium. Responding to my experiences, she states: "You have to train; all these experiences, all these feelings – you have to learn how to deal with it. Many people go through difficult experiences, and the only way to deal with them is to study and learn how to control them" (Interview 28 Jan. 2016). I must clarify that I have not even come close to completing mediumship training but have participated in different sessions of several mediumship groups, having been sustainedly affected by the voices of spirits, mediums, and other participants I had the opportunity to listen to.

Voices of Good Sense

Every society provides practices to reorganize their members' sensory worlds (Porcello et al. 2010; Downey 2016), for example, in religious-spiritual and/ or healing practices. Zarrilli (2015) argues that specific sensory-experiential worlds can be accessed by long-term and in-depth practices such as, for example, meditation. He detects attention, sensory awareness, and affect/ feeling as major achievement factors and forms of inner movement and experience. Accordingly, specific bodily practices and related embodied processes trigger transitions from one state of consciousness to another. Howes (2015), in this regard, mentions "techniques of the senses" as involved in the neural and mental organization of selves in their relation to specific environments. He provides an insightful example of Quakers "listening to silence," an aspect I will further explore and integrate with my interpretation of Spiritist practices:

> The apparent absence of (external) ritual and stimuli in general is tied to the privileging of the 'inner life' [...]. [W]e can begin to see how the very emphasis on the curtailment of the senses institutes a sensory regime in which 'silence' takes on positive qualities instead of simply denoting an absence and opens the individual to the most infinitesimal sensation – the quickening of the spirit.
>
> (Howes 2015: 161)

The reduction of external sensory stimuli to support internal reflection and adaption also appears to be crucial for discussing the Aesthetics of Healing in Brazilian Spiritist mental healthcare practices. Sensory anthropologists argue that within the alleged hierarchy of the senses from sight over sound, touch, taste down to smell in "Western" cultures, a stimulating shift from visual toward auditory perception would not just enable to more consciously explore "soundscapes" but help people to detract, relax, and engage with their "inner self." For the context of Brazilian religious practices, Rabelo et al. (2009) outline the importance of "cultivating the senses" through bodily engagement and the attunement to place (ibid.: 1f). They suggest exploring which sensory capacities are awakened and cultivated in a religious setting and how they frame embodied patterns of attention to self and others:

> A focus on place, or rather on our engagement with/in place, allows analysis to move from considering the senses as variables or factors acting to produce an experience toward approaching them as already enmeshed and articulated in a total experience – as 'praxis' that is both an exploration of place and response to the many summons of place. There is a fundamental reversibility between perception and the body's engagement in place, between sensing and moving [...].
>
> (Rabelo et al. 2009: 3)

As Rabelo et al. discuss concerning religious experience, I assess sensory modes in therapeutic spaces as crucial for their comprehension, especially at the intersection of religious/spiritual and medical interventions. Bodily engagement in religious/spiritual settings motivates efforts of self-transformation by cultivating sensibilities and body practices (ibid.: 6f).

Sound experience and the acquisition of a style of speech may play an important role here (ibid.: 11f), and even though the authors refer to Pentecostal practices, their observations also apply to Spiritism. The difference is that, at least in my personal experience, Pentecostal communities tend to engage in yells and loud utterances when allegedly speaking in angel's tongues, exorcising demons, or integrating Christian rock music performances into their services. In Kardecism, on the contrary, as far as it concerns my observations, listening to lectures, learning to lecture, and discussing the literature as methods of silent incorporation of knowledge seem to be at the core of well-being production. It not only differs from the boisterous Evangelical sermons or the performances of Afro-Brazilian practices with their costumes, food, masks, rhythms, dances, and chants (cf. Kurz 2013); it also appears to contradict the general loudness of everyday Brazilian life as I perceive it. Kardecism seems to intentionally counteract common cultural patterns of sensory expression by obtaining – at first sight – a certain passiveness of their clients, who appear to relax in a calm environment and turn to themselves. In my experience, entering Spiritist spaces always soothed me by providing (1) a cool shelter from the hot environment, (2) a quiet space as a refuge from noisy surroundings, and (3) attention in terms of listening and caring. Interaction and perception are widely reduced to low conversations and listening to the voices of lecturers and mediums/spirits.

With these observations in mind, I am convinced that even though they appear to create disengagement from any sensory engagement, working with senses is central to Spiritism: the unusual practice of passively listening in combination with extended monotonous lectures of variously skilled presenters mesmerizing their audience supports a state of exploring an inner self and the reflection of experiences. The practice of *passe* serves as a further strategy of bodily experience and reflection, and the consumed, allegedly fluidized water is the final act of internalization. Participants step back, listen, embody, and enact Spiritist ideals of self-care by caring for others. Volunteers repeatedly perform lectures at HEM, and with time, I observe differences in their performances and skills. Most talk with a friendly, warm, and soothing voice in a slow, flowing rhythm, using relatively simple language to attract their listeners' attention. Only once did a volunteer reach such a high pitch comparable to Pentecostal preachers, leaving the audience restless and confused.

Speaking skills are trained within study groups at HEM and CELV, where participants read aloud and comment on Spiritist literature, exercise to improvise spontaneous prayers and learn to integrate repeated formulas and quotes into their communication. Volunteers like Regina also make use of these techniques within the Evangelization meetings at HEM, and psychiatric inpatient Elisângela serves as an example of a person who internalizes what she listens to: she repeats her gained new knowledge whenever possible and feels responsible for passing it on to others. As most of my case studies in Chapter 3 reveal, sustained healing experiences only take place if afflicted persons continuously participate in lectures and study groups and start to develop agency as lecturers, group organizers, or advisors in fraternal care themselves. Regina, for example, provides space for the patients of HEM to reflect on and discuss Spiritist knowledge. Some patients like Elisângela extensively use it and relate to their situation what has been said. Others act differently and question everything said, sometimes having Regina lose her spirit. One of these skeptics is André, a highly educated young man with fluent English skills and broad philosophical and religious-spiritual knowledge. He is diagnosed with drug-induced psychosis, is convinced that everybody should have magic mushrooms to experience "real spirituality," and permanently disturbs the conversation for the sake of developing a "higher level of truth." In his opinion, participants are too simple-minded, and the whole discussion would not lead anywhere. Accordingly, Spiritist sessions may also bear internal conflicts, and this situation even escalates to the point that Regina's Spiritist habit of being a caring and loving person is challenged: André insists that people can learn something from him and that everybody should "shut up" and listen to his insights. Not being used to such resistance and criticism, Regina, a school teacher by profession, can hardly perform anymore, becomes agitated, and leaves in a nervous and powerless state after a quick *passe* and the Lord's Prayer. On our way out of the ward, she turns to me, saying: "What can drugs do? What was that? This lad is intelligent, and some things he said were exciting, but he is disturbed and full of negative energy. He should *learn to listen!*" (Session 25 Nov. 2015).

Apart from the fact that Regina is incapable of cognitively dealing with a situation that questions her embodied schemes and knowledge, her despaired outburst that people must "learn to listen" is remarkable. Kapchan (2009) investigates processes of "learning to listen" with an example of Sufism in France. She explores how sound encodes "sacred affect" and how it is trained (ibid.: 65). She observes that even though participants do not understand the meaning of recited texts, they acknowledge the "power of sound" and claim that it is about "spiritual audition" (ibid.: 66). It is a comparable example of "mimetic reproduction" (ibid.: 67) that does not necessarily aim at cognitive but mainly to sensory shifts within the audience, as it appears to be the case in Spiritist engagement at HEM and CELV, too. Kapchan differentiates divergent forms of listening and argues that learning to listen in Sufism is conceived as "listening with your heart," that is an active, attentive, and "deep" listening as an entire sensate being, a form of listening that ultimately induces trance (ibid.: 67). Obviously, when addressing the concept of "listening," we do not perceive it as a passive experience such as "hearing." What is essential is that there are different modes of active engagement with what is heard. Kapchan discusses how different ways or techniques of listening structure perception (ibid.: 67f) and observes that, for example, extended time frames of "structured silence" and "ritualized text reading and prayer" (ibid.: 71) play a significant role here, the same way I have outlined for Spiritist practices. Places transform into acoustic spaces that cultivate a specific affective stance and habitus of participants in relation to self, others, and environment (ibid.: 81).

Relating these theoretical insights to my ethnographic data, I argue that the reduction of stimuli to acoustic sensations and the practice of listening are essential to Spiritist mental healthcare. It is the calm and quiet nature that promotes a radical contrast to a noisy environment where other sensations more intensely occupy human perception, such as visual aesthetics, pleasant smell, or smooth body performance (see Chapter 2). I do not intend to generalize "Brazilian" sensory schemes, which is impossible due to the size and diversity of the country and its inhabitants. Attempts to explore "Brazilian sensory schemes and codings" reduce to small-scale environments and often focus on Afro-Brazilian (cf. Leibing 1995; van de Port 2005; Rabelo et al. 2009) or Indigenous (cf. Classen 1993, 1999) social groups. However, a more general attempt to explore Brazilian sensory worlds by Laplantine (2015) corresponds with my personal experience that the practice of "listening" usually is not reducible to "passive" attention but instead includes active engagement such as commenting and interrupting a speaker for the sake of "adding up to the story." This practice, which to me as a person socialized in Germany displays an impolite lack of basic social behavior, appears to be a common way of interaction for many Brazilians: certain news or narratives are "translated" into a shared experience that integrates cognitive message with affects and bodily engagement. In the very sense of the word, information is "shared" and negotiated. The negative effect is that few can narrate their entire stories. It is quite different in Spiritist environments, and I am convinced that it is a crucial experience for people in distress to experience an environment where they can express themselves, developing a sense of self apart from common procedures and practices that, in some cases, even are representing the causes of their affliction. It does not appear that individuals actively seek this alternative sensory environment, but Spiritist practices enhance capacities of active listening, irrespective of whether they are lecturers, discussants, instructors, mediums, or spirits. Accordingly, listening to voices becomes the focus of sensory experience, and this shift of sensory attention triggers a sixth sense of Self and Others.

Voices as ephemeral mediums of social and spiritual interaction and interconnection frame and shape participants' perceptions and how "social identities are represented, performed, transformed, evaluated, and contested" (Keane 2000: 271). Kolesch and Krämer (2006: 11f) underline the quality of voice as a performative phenomenon in multiple perspectives: it is an event when perceived by others at a specific moment; it may be a display of the relationship of actor and recipient; it involves embodiment of social relations and experience in the speaker and recipient; it carries the potential for subversion and transgression by transmission of unexpected meaning or distraction by uncontrolled bodily/sensory/emotional aspects which interfere with the message. Furthermore, voices are intersubjective as they promote interaction, sociability, communication, and positioning. They are liminal as they are sensual and senseful, physical and psychological, including action and reception, agency, and patiency. Voice is the experienced presence of an available or perhaps unavailable Other (ibid.: 12). Dolar (2006: 4) adds that listening to voices does not only include the grasping of a certain meaning or interaction but that the voice as such affects listeners. Voices have an aesthetic dimension: it is not about what is said but how it is said and how the recipient reacts to it (ibid.: 14). In opposition to written text, voices integrate individual markers such as accent, intonation, timbre, and personal performance style (ibid.: 20f). Voices break the silence, yet silence can also invoke internal voices heard by no one else (ibid.: 13f). Voices embody a passing presence (ibid.: 36) and affect us most intimately (ibid.: 40). In particular, hypnotic voices and ritually repeated formulas affect individuals on a deeper level and can create experiences of symbiosis between Self and Other (ibid.: 40f). Voices link meaning to bodily experience (ibid.: 59) and connect the internal Self with the external Other (ibid.: 71). Voices thus interact with our bodily capacities of sensory perception, cognition, and knowledge (Wagner-Egelhaaf 2017: 15).

Discussing voices at the intersection of psychiatric and Spiritist mental healthcare obtains an implicit level of meaningful experience when differentiating between voices of humans, spirits, and/or voices nobody else can listen to. Dein and Littlewood (2007), in this regard, discuss the experience of hearing voices as embedded in socio-cultural normalities, individual religious experiences, and medical evaluations. Their crucial insight is that religious-spiritual framings of the experience of listening to voices help avoid psychiatric treatments and encourage engagement with and exploration of these perceptions instead of avoidance or oppression. In this regard, Basu (2017a) addresses the intersection of religious and mental health practices and the question of to what extent symptoms of "hearing voices" might relate to insanity and/or religious-spiritual connotations. For the example of India, she stresses the quality of the voice as a medium of multidimensional sensory experience, emotional articulation (ibid. 2017b), and the importance of acousmatic (disembodied) voices in possession, illness, and healing rituals:

> The voice is a fugitive incident simultaneously appearing in the act of hearing and performance. The performance qualities of the voice, which appeal, compel, and evoke emotions, contribute to creating a 'sensuous geography' of the beyond through possession healing. Places, bodies, and selves become linked through the sense of hearing.
>
> (Basu 2017b: 260f)

Accordingly, voices are central performative agents in mediumistic healing rituals of possession (ibid.: 263). Healing practices unfold a soundscape of multiple voices, and spirits become tangible with the materialization of voices (ibid.: 264), as is the case in Spiritist disobsession practices. In particular, Basu (2014b) directs her attention toward different meanings of "hearing disembodied voices" in religious and psychiatric contexts. She explores the reception of related experiences in vernacular and psychiatric conceptions of pathology, ritual, and practices of care, pointing out that the experience of "hearing voices" might not be a symptom but a resource of healing madness: "Hearing disembodied voices figures importantly in the clinical picture of the syndrome of schizophrenia. In states of trance, however, hearing disembodied voices is considered a normal experience" (Basu 2014b: 327). At the intersection of psychiatric and religious-spiritual explanatory models on the experience of listening to (disembodied) voices, Basu stresses their performative and sensory aspects bridging self and other, inside and outside:

> The voice is performative, at once appealing, compelling and evoking emotions. The topology of the voice transcends dualisms, failing to correspond to 'Western' dualistic thought. [...] [N]otions of madness related to possession and sorcery draw on dual conceptions of embodied and disembodied minds, or 'mind-powers' [...] which are transcended in trance by the medium of the voice.
>
> (Basu 2014b: 329)

Basu (2018) argues that practices of spirit possession, mediumship, and related experiences of listening to voices should be understood as practices of knowledge, memory, healing, and an alternative theory of "madness" that stresses the transgressions in relationships of exchange between human and non-human agents. In the context of Spiritism, different categories of voices as media of interaction gain importance in particular practices and situations: throughout the fraternal care and lectures, the voices of volunteers (many having been patients and now are healers) are predominant. In mediumship sessions, the voices of participants, mediums (most of them, in a way, being patients and healers simultaneously), and spirits (some are patients, some are healers) predominate. Reminiscent of Latour (cf. 1996), I thus observe that the categories of patients, healers, mediums, spirits, and caretakers become blurred and reveal networks of agencies interconnected by voices. Therefore, our focus should not be so much on who is saying something for what purpose but on what it does to the listeners. Consequently, it is not about the transported messages but the reception and reaction of listeners. In Spiritism, the affective arrangement (cf. Slaby et al. 2017) of voices produces alternate states of awareness, consciousness, and perception, and in mediumship training, related techniques and skills are developed. They aim at human sensory qualities and capacities that establish, cultivate, elaborate, and utilize a "sixth sense" to benefit (self-)care.

Sixth Sense?!

Howes (2009) discusses religious-spiritual practices as capacities to cultivate a "sixth sense"[1] to (re)organize and (re)frame experiences of Self and Other. So far, it has remained obscure what exactly the sensory modalities and techniques are that shape the alleged transformation of experience and self-perception in mediumship training and the cultivation of an inner sense and/or interoceptive processes within Spiritist practices. Crabtree (2015: 11), in this regard, refers to the concept of a "subliminal self" as an aspect of the human psyche that usually is not accessible to consciousness but unravels in extraordinary situations such as dreams, hypnosis, paranormal experiences, or dissociative states (ibid.: 20). He wonders if mediumship might be a portal to enter this subliminal state and to consciously process and regulate interoceptive stimuli and related effects (cf. Critchley & Garfinkel 2017). Mediums in Marília narrate that they perceive surrounding spirits with all their senses: some see, some hear, some smell, feel, or even taste them. Often, it is a synesthetic experience of several senses and feelings, such as fatigue, nervousness, indefinite pain, anxiety, sadness, and/or disgust. As my vignettes in the previous (sub)chapters suggest, the audience of mediumship practices, including myself, also become affected by the experience and are guided toward some innovative models to perceive themselves in relation to "Others."

To further investigate the techniques and experiences of developing such a sixth sense, I turn to Classen (1999) and Pink (2009), who suggest integrating the researchers' sensory perceptions as data and comparing them to the interlocutors' narratives and interpretations. I am aware of the challenges and pitfalls such an approach might bear (see Chapter 1), but I am convinced that I can only understand mediumship practices by reflecting on *my* perceptions in the light of *their* explanations: listening to the mediums' voices and the spirits' narratives caused intense shifts of feelings between fright, empathy, and pity in me. Sometimes, the form and content of transmitted messages would be revealed to me by gut feelings, experiences of sudden anger, or tears running down my face even before being communicated by mediums. As I have already indicated, several times, I caught myself crying, being angry, devastated, or even feeling somatic pain for no apparent reason within these sessions, just to afterward listen to the spirits' messages corresponding to these sensations. What increasingly has become evident to me is that Spiritist practices do not simply develop techniques to access altered states of sensory perception[2] but that, particularly in mediumship training, the emphasis is on learning how to control and use them. Just as a newborn child must learn to process, distinguish, and interrelate what it sees, hears, tastes, smells, touches and is trained to evaluate sensory perceptions, mediums pass what we might call a second socialization of sensory perception.

Isabel went through similar experiences and has participated in Magali's mediumship training group for over four years. She is 53 years old, married, has two children and one granddaughter, and works in a lawyer's office. She has visited CELV for over 20 years since suffering from severe depression and panic attacks in 1994. She underwent unsuccessful psychiatric treatment until her psychotherapist suggested that she attend a Spiritist center. She took the advice and found relief in fraternal care with its affiliated lectures and subsequent study groups of Spiritist doctrine (see Chapter 3). After some time, she was asked to become an orienteer herself, for only those who have defeated depression could help others with similar conditions. She began working on her mediumship skills and learned to support others by sharing her experiences. She states that

[w]ith time, I increasingly noticed symptoms of mediumship in myself, like crying out of the blue for no reason, even about television advertisements for sanitary products, but also having visions of terrible things happening. I told Magali, and she convinced me to start working on my mediumship, that depression would be a common symptom. From then on, I started to participate in her medium training group to see what would happen, and then she made me direct another group because it was an issue of training and development for both the mediums and the instructors. It requires much studying because it is all about knowledge. [...] We must learn how to interact with people.

(Interview 26 Jan. 2016)

It becomes apparent how Spiritists integrate psychiatric discourse but transform, convert, and reframe it: depression is a symptom of mediumship and not vice versa. Treatment does not address a recovery back to normal but allows the (re)learning of how to interact with people, perform in certain situations, and deal with feelings and emotions. Isabel states that this transformation works mainly in terms of *reforma intima* ("inner reform"), meaning that persons must reflect on their issues and behavior in spiritual, energetical, and karmic terms. Throughout several courses, she learned about spiritual obsessors and how they affect human beings in terms of behavioral deviance, personal issues, and (mental) health problems.

In a further step, retired high school teacher Wilson integrates developing mediums in his mediumship training sessions that prepare mediums of CELV to participate in disobsession meetings at HEM to detect hostile spiritual agencies that affect patients or the hospital as an institution. I have participated in that group, too. At first sight, it seems that his training focuses on the cognitive internalization of Spiritist knowledge, but it is just another example of how voices and "formulas" of constantly repeated messages evoke altered states of sensory perception. His mediumship training and disobsession meetings occur thrice a week on Monday and Tuesday evenings and on Saturday mornings and usually last one to two hours. Like all the previously described sessions, they reveal a ritualistic structure even though participants stress that they do not perform rituals but apply techniques. In a plain, undecorated room, 10–20 persons of different ages and genders sit around a table. Upon arrival, participants greet the others and converse while writing their names and those of patients or people they wish to support into a textbook. Wilson then calls for silence and asks each participant to read out psychographic messages from past meet-ings. Their continuous repetition seems to serve as a means of incorporating knowledge and transforming an idea into a habit. It appears as an eternal loop of repeated messages without significant content: "The divine master loved and protected, fought in favor of light, resisted the shadows until the cross, and we are here on earth to learn and help." Another idiom would be: "When the struggle displeases, love comes into sight; against light and charity, darkness cannot persist." I have wondered how these platitudes are meant to produce insight or resolve personal issues. However, they seem essential in transforming participants' perceptions regarding therapeutic and self-healing capacities of Spiritist engagement. Wilson continues with prayers "in the name of love and charity" for the spiritual support and protection of explicitly named community members, patients, and staff of HEM. Subsequently, several participants read out loud selected passages from Kardec's "Mediums' Book" (1986) or other spontaneously selected texts Wilson deems crucial for the education and discipline of mediums. To me, the ever-repeated message is that thoughts, feelings, and our ways of talking must be trained because thoughts influence reality, and words affect our thoughts, feelings, health, and personal development. Throughout the lectures, others provide *passe* to the group, and I often observe changes in body posture, tension, and emanation in myself and other participants.

The doors are locked, and the room is darkened; this is when "the work" is initiated: the names and addresses of afflicted or deceased persons are read aloud, and a commentary on their affliction is given in an endless loop of prayer that stimulates concentration and release in waves: Wilson prays for a person and then falls into silence. Then, another group member mentions another name, which is discussed until Wilson returns to his mantra-like prayer to integrate these persons into his evocation. I perceive the develop-ment of a certain rhythm of different voices and phases of silence, which blur my observer's, or better, listener's, mind, leaving me dizzy. Then again, there is silence until someone initiates another invocation, followed by the Lord's Prayer. Suddenly, some of the participants start sighing, moaning, yawning, and shivering. Others hold their head in their hands, almost passing out. People sense strange vibrations, receive messages, or even incorporate spirits and are told by Wilson to recite the Lord's Prayer. As a participant, I cannot listen to everything, but I am aware of a murmuring of mixed voices. As in previous sessions, my shoulders feel heavy. Vera, one of the orienteers, comes to give me a *passe* and tells me to recite the Lord's Prayer. She continues with another prayer to "resolve this situation" and tells me to call her whenever I feel something. Vera and Wilson act like this with all the participants, partaking in the others' impressions, feelings, and visions and supporting their self-discipline through prayer.

Some participants transmit messages of spirits' death or afterlife experiences. They often express affection or vengeful feelings toward a particular person, thus causing affliction. The spirits are thought to be obsessors of HEM patients, people who had already been prayed for, or even session participants. Wilson and Vera initiate conversations with all of them, and after some minutes of resistance, the conversation usually results in the same way: the spirits give in and acknowledge their adverse action against themselves and others. They are guided by helping spirits to the hospital on a higher spiritual level (see Chapter 3), where they may progress spiritually, reunite with family members or friends, and prepare for the next incarnation. Some cases seem dramatic, but I can only hear low voices, sobbing, and sighing. I am not comprehending the stories and start to take a sensory dive into this buzzing and bubbling of voices. I like this feeling, and it would carry me away if it were not for Wilson, who relays a supposedly important psychographic message that another participant had just produced: "In this house of Jesus, we have some problems that we can only resolve with his blessings: stasis, discouragement, and adversity." Everybody must repeat this insight several times aloud, first together, then separately, one after another. Things begin returning to normal, and the session is concluded by giving thanks and reciting the Lord's Prayer, and the idioms read aloud at the beginning of the session are revisited once again (Session 01 Dec. 2015).

Here, we witness another quality of voices: they not only trigger certain inner sensory perceptions but can also redirect attention to the external environment. The different voices found in lectures, prayers, mediumistic messages, and orientations guide the participants through altered states of sensory perception without losing contact and track of "reality."[3]

I have participated in these sessions every week, and – as I have indicated – with time, it has done something to me. A few weeks after my first disobsession meeting with Wilson, I keep my eyes closed for almost the entire session. Even though I sit in an uncomfortable chair and position, I perceive a soothing relaxation taking shape within me, followed by waves of heaviness and lightness streaming through my body, bringing me to support my head with my hands so as not to crash into the table. I "see" a blue field that disappears into blackness. This "black hole" then transforms into a white light, which is not simply there but stays pulsating for several minutes.

I perceive it as beautiful and think of *chakras* as centers of energetic transmission. I see the blue field return before it slowly dissolves. Then I "wake up" and notice that I have hardly heard anything said during this session. Reluctantly, others describe similar impressions, and medium Lucia explains that this has been a collective *passe* for all of us by "higher" benevolent spirits. This episode occurred before my previously described accounts, but I refer to it here to stress how sensory perceptions are triggered and how I, as a *gringo*, have developed an increasing attunement to them. From this incident onward, I wanted to learn more about the importance of sensory perception, attunement, and discipline of "fellow" mediums.

Being regular participants of Wilson's Saturday morning mediumship session, I became friends with the couple Liliane and Bruno. Liliane is 31 years old and an accountant; Bruno is 35 and a legal administrator. One evening, they invite me to their house to participate in their private *Evangelho no Lar* ("Gospels at Home"), reading and discussing Spiritist literature with family members and friends, followed by a long conversation on our perceptions and interpretations of mediumship practices. Liliane tells me that since she was a young girl, she would see spirits and other "strange things." The first instance she remembers was when she was four years old and woke up at night, watching her doll moving and waving with her eyes blinking. Her devoted Catholic mother would not believe her reports, pushing them away as imagination. Since then, "things would happen," sometimes in a very subtle way, even hard to grasp, but it would leave her frightened. By the age of seven, the family moved to another house, and she started to regularly see a blond girl at the door to her room. Whenever she would fall asleep, she would hear steps but could not locate their source. Liliane declares that she lived in continuous fear and affliction in this house, but nobody would believe her. Her father even took her to a psychiatrist who "diagnosed" that she was asking for attention but still wanted to assign her to HEM and prescribed strong tranquilizers. Her parents resisted but also did not seek alternative support until one day, a neighbor told her father that years ago, a convicted murderer had lived in that house and that he had killed at least one of his victims in this house. At least by that point, her parents would take her observations more seriously but still did not know how to resolve the problem. Some years after moving in, her father began reforming the house and found finger-nails and hair between the bricks when tearing down a wall.[4] Fearful of what else he might find, but without any resources to move out, he stopped the enterprise and called several priests of divergent Christian denominations to bless and "cleanse" the house. The family lived there for another 10 years, and "things" continued to happen: she heard footsteps, doors opened without any traceable cause, and sometimes she would see "that girl." Even a dog her parents gave her as a companion would refuse to enter the house, apparently being as frightened as she was. It took all of this for her parents to accept that something "really wrong" was going on, and

> [f]inally, after all these years, my Mum turned to Spiritism, after calling priests from various churches to bless, but nothing would work out. We met this guy from a Spiritist center, and in my ignorance, I thought we would have to go there once, and then the problem would be resolved. We stayed there for a lecture, but, of course, nothing was resolved. We started to frequent regularly, but nothing would change at home, and we stopped going.
>
> (Interview 13 Dec. 2015)

Years later, after she had started dating Bruno, who at the time already was a practicing Spiritist, she began to frequent CELV again, engaging as a volunteer at HEM and "working" as a medium. Bruno reports that his story is less dramatic but that he and an aunt would have had healing experiences regarding chronic somatic distress at Spiritist centers. For this reason, he started engaging with Spiritism and even developed the "subtle mediumistic skill of psychography" while participating in Wilson's group since 2012. Liliane continues that from the beginning, the lectures and studies supported her in reflecting on her situation, but her most significant improvement came after refining her mediumship skills. It helps her to "release some pressure" by communicating her perceptions but also to see the condition of psychiatric patients who, parallel to their Saturday meetings, listen to the morning lecture and afterward receive the *passe* from them and their fellow participants, leaving her to feel more humble and thankful for what she has. She admits that she still must learn to be more patient and tolerant with "others" and that it is something that she tries to cultivate every day a little bit more. The more she engages in it, the less she will have disturbing experiences. She still perceives "the deceased" every single day and feels the urge to communicate, but only within the sessions does she experience the framework to do so:

> I am not the kind of medium who sees and can interact. It is more like flashes or phrases that appear but not in a way you can directly help. However, once I decided to help them, I had to do it there [at HEM]. Maybe you already noticed that I often start saying things like last week, I perceived this and that. I saw something, listened to something, had a dream, felt bad, etc., and then I arrive there, and it makes me feel better. I believe they are helped, but I go because it makes me feel good. It is weird: I am conscious of what I say and of what I feel, and it feels as if it is me. The pain I feel seems to be my pain, this anger, this anxiety, this despair. I think I need help, but then Pedro [another orienteer] usually shows up, and I can put it out. After it passed, I see that it was not me but somebody else.
>
> (Interview 13 Dec. 2015)

Liliane continues by reporting that after the sessions, she usually feels hungry and tired but that during the day, especially after having a shower, changing clothes, and perhaps having a nap, she feels much better. She must go every week, or else she would remain in bad shape, suffering from headaches, insomnia, and perceiving things happening in the house: "I see and hear things; the bed stays shaking while Bruno sleeps like a bear." Bruno confirms that when they do not go every week, he also feels sensations of heaviness, laziness, tiredness, stress, or nervousness. He is convinced it is due to spirits still connected to "the material existence" and, therefore, seek links to interact. In the mediumship sessions, participants would try to treat and resolve this harmful affection:

> You come with that heaviness, and you leave as being renovated, easy, light, happy, recharged; and especially after giving *passe* to the patients because it is not only about our energy but the spiritual one, and we are only transmitters. This is good for us and them simultaneously: of course, we perceive this disturbed ambient over there, but helping them is helping us feel better afterward.
>
> (Interview 13 Dec. 2015)

Selves and Others

Mauss (1975) addressed the human body as a socio-cultural matrix of self and personhood. Among others, Douglas (1970), Scheper-Hughes and Lock (1987), and Csordas (1990) have further developed this approach to investigate divergent categories of Self and Other and the ways in which humans use their bodies in socio-cultural contexts, cosmologies, ideologies, and/or fashions. Mauss introduced concepts relevant to our discussion, such as body techniques and habitus, the latter being further elaborated by Bourdieu (1977), and the former by Foucault (1988b) in terms of "technologies of the self." These concepts are crucial for comprehending the Aesthetics of Healing in Spiritism in terms of developing a (sixth?) sense of Self and Other. I have elaborated on how Spiritist healing practices can be regarded as bodily/sensory techniques to generate a specific habitus and how certain technologies of the self may trigger and/or control sensory perceptions at the margin of what is deemed "normal" experience and behavior in Brazil. Black (2018), in this regard, outlines the importance of communicative processes that constitute practices of (self-)care, agency, and creativity, emphasizing the relationality of caregivers and caretakers and moral-ethical frames of the relationship with others and oneself as social practices and embodied experience. Cognitive scientist Gibbs (2005) similarly argues that any communication is embodied (inter)action and that our body is the medium to communicate with the world (ibid.: 14f). However, he questions a strict self-environment-dualism of independent categories and instead, reminiscent of Varela et al. (1999), suggests the perspective of a self-environment-mutuality that is enacted (Gibbs 2005: 16f). Noland (2009), in his survey on embodiment and agency, stresses the importance of bodily/sensory techniques for these ends, and Hume (2007) even speaks of the senses as portals to open doorways to other realities, ways of interaction, and forms of healing. Her manifold examples of sensory manipulation in religious-spiritual and healing practices illustrate that there are veritable technologies to generate altered states of consciousness (ASC) or, as I prefer to label it, altered states of sensory perception (ASSP).

My accounts on mediumship practices and several participants' narratives reveal insights on ASSP: (1) they may occur at the intersection of brain activities, for example on the edge of being awake and falling asleep (see the examples of Liliane in the previous subchapter and Regina in Chapter 3), (2) they are triggered, controlled, and transformed in settings where shifts of sensory perception are produced, and (3) conventional psychiatry tends to oppress these perceptions and experiences, whereas, in Spiritism, they are valued and shared to help others. For the latter reason, at HEM and the affiliated CELV, they are integrated into practices of (self-)care. Moreover, the accounts of my observations and personal experiences reveal how the reduction of sensory stimuli and the practice of listening to voices provide a space that simultaneously sensitizes for inner processes and transforms participants' experiences and interpretations of external and environmental dynamics. The Aesthetics of Healing in Spiritist mental healthcare consist of several interventions and performative arrangements, cognitive acquisition and embodiment, sensory triggering and control, and the development of a spiritual habitus that negotiates experiences of Self and Other. Liliane, for example, highlights her claim that Spiritist practice helps her be more patient and tolerant with others, that is, psychiatric patients at HEM *and* their obsessing spirits, and Bruno confirms that it is "good for them and us." More than that, their experiences reveal a model of agency that is worth further exploring in medical anthropology: in Spiritist mediumship practices, humans do not appear to use spirits for their purposes (e.g., in terms of sorcery or witchcraft), but spirits make use of the human sensorium to interact and produce a temporary space for *their* well-being. These ideas are based on a concept of person or self that is not grounded in the assumption of a closed, autonomous entity (individual), nor exclusively being defined through the relations to others, including spirits or ancestors: the Self in Spiritism negotiates between these aspects and agencies. Spiritist volunteers and especially the mediums engage with the Others (both patients and obsessors) with a sense of empathy. Liliane's case reveals her efforts to do so, and all the other case studies discussed in this and the previous chapters also support the idea that at least one capacity to be triggered and developed in Spiritist practice is a sense of empathy with others.

Skultans (2007) has described comparable experiences among Spiritualists in Wales as empathy in a twofold way: illness is interpreted as socio-somatic, and social attention resolves the problem, and second, participants learn to see the aura of a person and by this develop understanding and empathy. Hollan and Throop (2008) declare empathy a little explored concept in anthropology, also due to Geertz's (1974) criticism that it would only apply to a "Western" individualistic understanding of self and person. However, as Eller (2019: 117f) puts it, the categories of "individual" and "dividual" personhood are artificial, and in different cultural and social contexts, the Self would identify as a hybrid of both. Therefore, Hollan and Throop (2008: 385f) guess that humans generally develop a concern with what motivates others, and every culture provides resources to enable and suppress capacities to build empathy for others. They attribute certain psychological states, shared feelings, or emotional attunement to this relation of Self and Other but are undecided if this is due to an imaginative projection from Self on Other or a veritable capacity of participation in other's feelings and ideas (ibid.: 386). The latter would undoubtedly apply to Spiritist practices, especially when we extend the concept of "Other" to spirits. In Spiritism, the delimitations of Self and Other are not entirely clear-cut due to a model of personhood that integrates a biological body, an immortal and reincarnating spirit, the *perispirit* as the bearer of karmic issues, and through the latter, relationships to living and deceased spirits. Hollan and Throop address this problem by stating that there might be differences in porous or impermeable boundaries of Self (ibid.: 389) but assume that in any case, intersubjective and intentional agencies imply sensory-based modes of knowing and a theory of mind of the other (ibid.: 386f). Accordingly, they define empathy as an ongoing, dialogical, intersubjective accomplishment.

We can undoubtedly consider Spiritist healing practices as a context where a sense of empathy is developed by simultaneously (re)defining what is "Self" and "Other." Explanatory models of obsession or mediumship externalize specific experiences but still must be dealt with in terms of care of Selves and Others (e.g., patients at HEM, clients at CELV, Spiritist volunteers, and spirits). Kirmayer's (2008) reports from clinical psychotherapy on how some experiences of radical otherness challenge the affective, communicative, and imaginative processes that underlie empathy applies very well to Liliane's statement that she tries every day to be a little bit more patient and tolerant with "them," that is, the Other. However, before being able to do so, she had to find out what is "hers" and what is "theirs." This is accomplished by a looping effect (cf. Hacking 1995) of self-reflection, causal understanding, change of habits, and again self-reflection. At some point in this spiral process, a Self or person feels different from what it was before. It is like a second socialization of sensory perception that, according to my interlocutor Taylor, includes the perception through the *perispirit* at the intersection of internal and external factors of Self and Otherness.

Whatever that "sixth sense" developed in Spiritist healing practices can be labeled (mediumship, empathy, or a sense of Self and Other), I am convinced that it implies first developing a "sense of self" in terms of the exploration of an "inner self" and, therefore, interoceptive capacities. Throughout this chapter, I have illustrated that Spiritist healing practices can be considered contemplative practices due to their structure and sensory arrangements. Downey (2015: 47f) relates contemplative practices to somatosensory and interoceptive processing and interprets them as practices of self-cultivation fostering self-comfort, self-manipulation, and self-shaping. Considering Ingold (2000) and his focus on the education of attention, Downey (2016: 48) stresses the importance of sensory skills and enculturation as a dynamic of perceptual learning. He argues that a sensory-based education of attention as a way of cultural learning is more substantial and easily embodied than any cognitive system of learning (ibid.: 48). Sensory learning, thus, is a form of enculturation and bodily practice that opposes the image of rationally internalized cognitive schemes as we might expect when taking into consideration the reading and study aspect of Spiritist practice. However, it is not just about cognitive comprehension of the Spiritist doctrine; the various episodes of lecture, prayer, and silence are techniques to produce, control, and shape an internal sensory perception, that is, interoception and mediumship. This does not mean that mediumship would not relate to external agents like spirits, but the skill of mediumship is the capacity to direct the medium's perception to internal stimuli. Farb et al. (2015) conceptualize interoception as the sensory perception of stimuli produced within the body and perceive it as central to any form of embodiment, motivation, and well-being. In particular, Asian mindfulness practices, with their theories of a subtle body (similar to the concept of the *perispirit*), would pay more attention to the body and internal processes. Conceptualizing body and self as being exposed to positive and negative energies of the universe, they would aim at (re)directing the body toward the "right tracks." The authors also present some examples of successful integration of these concepts into psychotherapy, stressing the importance of transformation of self, perception, and self-perception (cf. Kabat-Zinn 2003; Kirmayer 2015). Even though I am critical of imposing certain cultural concepts on other contexts, I am convinced that Spiritist healing practices are comparable to these techniques as they aim to focus and control sensory perception instead of dissociation or distraction. Varela et al. (1999: 24f) argue that to understand mindfulness, one must realize that most people are not mindful. Usually, our mind wanders around, which, in the Buddhist sense, makes us "not present," or, as I want to add, not completely aware of ourselves and our presence in the world. Mindfulness trains two stages of practice: first, calming the mind, and second, the development of insight. The purpose of calming the mind is not to become absorbed but to render the mind able to be present with itself long enough to gain insight into its nature and functioning (ibid.: 25f). My experiences of Spiritist healing practices apply to this model: they strengthen specific modes of (sensory) attention and provide techniques not to become distracted, as is evident in Wilson's mediumship sessions. In this regard, Varela et al.'s discussion provides support for my method of integrating personal sensory experiences with the analysis of Spiritist mental healthcare:

> The meditator now discovers that the abstract attitude that Heidegger and Merleau-Ponty ascribe to science and philosophy is actually the attitude of everyday life when one is not mindful. This abstract attitude is the spacesuit, the padding of habits and preconceptions, the armor with which one habitually distances oneself from one's experience. From the point of view of mindfulness/awareness meditation, humans are not trapped forever in the abstract attitude. The dissociation of mind from body, of awareness from experience, is the result of habit, and these habits can be broken.
>
> (Varela et al. 1999: 25)

It is what I have tried to do with my autoethnographic accounts on Spiritist healing practices: transgressing regular perceptive patterns of participant observation and observational participation and instead diving into the sensory universe of practice, becoming aware of it, making sense out of it, and only then interpreting it in comparison with my interlocutors' narratives instead of imposing pre-modeled patterns of cognitive abstraction. It is not an attempt to substitute "common" ethnography, nor does it negate the value of abstraction, comparison, and evaluation; it rather is a complement to meet and comprehend the experiences of the people involved thoroughly. Wallace (2012) confirms this aspect of mindfulness and introspection as a method to explore practices of Spiritst mental healthcare:

> Therefore the refinement of attention is of universal relevance. It involves training two faculties: (1) one is mindfulness, the faculty of sustaining voluntary attention, continuously, upon a chosen object. [...] Mindfulness is an extraordinarily important faculty of the mind that can be refined [...] beyond anything that can be imagined by the scientific community, and (2) introspection is a faculty of monitoring the mind, direct observing states of consciousness, and other mental processes.
>
> (Wallace 2012: 162)

Training attention aims at cultivating a more profound sense of ease and relaxation in the mind–body and stability, continuity, and coherence of attention to a particular object. In the case of Kardecist mediumship, one must learn to focus on the inner senses and how to deal with specific, possibly afflicting sensations and perceptions. In summary, I conclude that by applying the theoretical model of Aesthetics of Healing, cultivating an inner sense in relation to "something other" is central to Spiritist healing practices and, in particular, to Kardecist mediumship training. Based on these insights, I am convinced these skills are related to sensory perception and comparable to mindfulness and interoception training practices. Spiritist healing practices focus on voices as sensory stimuli and provide sensory-bodily techniques to shift attention. Psychotherapists (cf. Kabat-Zinn 2003; Kirmayer 2015) have applied these concepts, and so should medical anthropologists in their discussion of sensory experiences in therapeutic contexts. The Aesthetics of Healing do not reduce to the (symbolic) communication or incorporation of external ideas and values but, on the contrary, link to the perception and experience of Self and Other. They surpass the notion of how our senses are manipulated in certain sensory arrangements by addressing how senses such as interoception, mediumship, and/or empathy are developed in processes of self-empowerment and (self-) awareness.

The fact that some elements of Spiritit healing practices appear to be comparable to Asian (Buddhist) concepts such as reincarnation, karma, chakras, energy fields and a subtle body, mindfulness and contemplation, interoception and self-awareness does not mean that I tend to equal them with each other. Even though Skultan's (2007) account of "aura-reading" in Welsh Spiritualism relates to contemporary discourses on chakras and energies in Brazilian Spiritism that appear to derive from Buddhist practice and discourse, I refuse any attempt of equation. We must investigate each practice in its own rights and contexts. However, comparison allows for discussing translocal and transcultural transfers and transformations of healing practices and their distribution as Complementary and Alternative Medicines (CAM) in different contexts. Chapter 5 will thus leave the local contexts of HEM and CELV and explore wider networks of Spiritism in Marília, Brazil, and beyond.

Notes

1 Like "seeing and hearing dead people" in the Hollywood blockbuster The Sixth Sense (Shyamalan 1999)?
2 Reminiscent of the concept of altered states of consciousness (ASC).
3 Similar qualities have been attributed to the chants of "shamans," especially regarding healing experiences (cf. Lévi-Strauss 1963; Brabec de Mori 2002, 2015).
4 It does not automatically indicate that somebody was "disposed" of but may also refer to common Brazilian ideas of *macumba* ("black magic" as related to Afro-Brazilian practices) to place a spell or curse.

Chapter 5

Translocal Networks and Politics of Care

Exploring divergent spaces of Spiritist (mental) healthcare in Brazil, in October 2011, I encountered a German doctor in Bahia. On a Thursday morning at 7 o'clock, my wife and I arrived at the Spiritist center *Porta de Esperança* ("Gateway to Hope") in Ilheus, getting in line with about 15 other persons and listening to an elderly woman's statement that over here, you must arrive early because Dr. Hans attracts many patients. However, arriving early does not mean being treated fast and leaving soon again. Quite the opposite, visitors gather in a waiting room with meditative music playing in the background. Some visitors chat quietly while others read Spiritist literature or enjoy the free coffee and bread. Two men lecture on love, charity, and health and speak some prayers. At 11 o'clock, free soup is shared with everybody. It appears like a social gathering if it were not for the visible symptoms of diverse afflictions many participants display. To me, it feels like waiting eternally without even knowing what exactly I am waiting for. At some point around noon, we are called to another room to receive a *passe* and learn that Dr. Hans and his team will soon attend us. However, it still takes another hour until we are called into a room with four psychologists who volunteer to perform an anamnesis and ask for our motivations to come here. I am directed to one of them and identify as an anthropologist, expressing my interest in learning more about health practices. I add that I have suffered for years from back pain that has not been cured so far. Besides stating that Lindomar, the medium of Dr. Hans, would be able to help me with my affliction, she promises that she would arrange a private meeting to learn more about the work of Dr. Hans/Lindomar. Whereas the latter has never happened, the former indeed occurs: we are finally called into the *sala mediunica* (mediumship hall), the actual treatment facility. Sitting in rows of plastic chairs, people receive a *passe* by Dr. Hans/Lindomar, and he calls some to lay on a stretcher, including me. I receive a brief massage, and I have to admit that ever since my back pain has diminished.[1] Upon leaving the site around 2 p.m., the psychologist briefly meets me again to ensure I understand that Dr. Hans was a German doctor who died in one of the World Wars.

DOI: 10.4324/9781032637167-5

My vignette displays a unique variant of healing cooperation that differs from *Hospital Espírita de Marília* (HEM) and *Centro Espírita Luz e Verdade* (CELV) in Marília: the interaction of human patients with discarnate medical professionals. It has been this branch of Brazilian Spiritism that attracted more attention from public media and science, particularly social anthropologists, due to cases of surgeries on the material body of patients without any anesthetic or hygienic precautions, e.g., by Dr. Fritz (Greenfield 2008) and John of God (Rocha 2017). Being legally sanctioned, most spirit doctors nowadays only treat the energetic-spiritual body of their patients. Like Dr. Fritz, most of them appear to be the spirits of German medical doctors who died in the World Wars and now engage in spiritual treatments through their Brazilian mediums. Many of my interlocutors explain this "fact" in one of these terms: (1) Spiritist knowledge originally derives from Germany (see Chapter 2), (2) many German medical doctors throughout the World Wars engaged in inhumane experiments and are now trying to pay off their karmic debts, and (3) being German to many Brazilians is a synonym for effectiveness. Within the Afro-Brazilian religion of *Umbanda*, spirits of formerly enslaved or Indigenous people act as spirit doctors, but throughout my research on Kardecist Spiritism, I mainly met "German" ones, such as Dr. Frederic (Vitória/Espírito Santo), Dr. Hans (Ilheus/Bahia), Dr. Hermann (Araraquara/São Paulo), and Dr. Wilhelm (Marília/São Paulo). However, I also engaged with Dr. Claudionor (Itabuna/Bahia), who, in his lifetime, had allegedly been a medical doctor in São Paulo. I guess that in performative terms, the example of Dr. Claudinor as an entity from the technologically advanced Southeast of Brazil acting in the less developed Northeast of Brazil resembles, in a way, the prejudice of Germans being more effective than Brazilians, that is, the idea of a spirit from technologically more advanced spheres supporting the disadvantaged. On the other hand, Rocha (2017) points out that the supposedly genuine Brazilian spirit of João de Deus ("John of God") mainly attracts "Western" patients from all over the world, seeking "the other" in "holistic" and/or "spiritual" therapies.

In the previous chapters, I have outlined how Spiritist practices establish Healing Cooperation between mental health professionals and religious/spiritual healers. Focusing on the Aesthetics of Healing, I have argued that it initiates perceptional reconfigurations and transformations regarding the sense of Self and Other. I have also indicated that, at the margin of the 21st century, Spiritism has not only had an increasing impact on the Brazilian mental healthcare provision but also abroad. Accordingly, in this chapter, I will disclose some implications of Spiritist networks regarding their health practices' implementation in different localities. I will introduce interrelated but diversified spaces of Spiritist (mental) healthcare by first moving from the center of Marília (São Paulo, Brazil; see Chapters 3 and 4) to its peripheries, then to its wider surroundings in the state of São Paulo, and further to the Northeastern state of Bahia which in political, economic, ethnic, and socio-cultural terms varies a great deal from the Southeast (cf. Kurz 2013). I will further expand my analysis of translocal networks of Kardecism in Brazil to their (re)implementation in Germany by Brazilian migrants, following some of my interlocutors' connections. I will discuss the negotiation of Spiritist practice and knowledge in the context of migration and appropriation with "locals" to investigate how agencies and practices interconnect on local, regional, national, and translocal/-national levels and, on the other hand, how they adapt to their respective environments and give voice to related experiences.

Translocal Spiritism Revisited

Rocha (2017) analyzes Spiritist healing practices in terms of a hypothetical contrast between "religion" and "spirituality" that would materialize in the shape of a global increase of "individual spirituality as personal transformation" opposing "social religiosity as a public institution" intertwining with a new global popular health culture (ibid.: 7; see Chapter 2). Research on so-called Complementary and Alternative Medicines (CAM) assumes conceptual hybridization and dissolution of ethnic, religious, or national boundaries (Ross 2012; Kirmayer 2015), but investigations regarding Brazilian Spiritism in translocal contexts illustrate heterogeneous dynamics: whereas Sterzi (2011) observes a close connection between Spiritist practice and diasporic identity and Brazilian migratory experience management in Great Britain, Saraiva (2010), for the example of Portugal, describes a melting pot and integration of different socio-cultural influences.

Considering these diverse dynamics, I decided to further explore the implementation of Spiritist mental healthcare practice in Germany for four reasons: (1) as outlined in Chapter 2, Germany can be considered a breeding ground of Spiritist thought and practice; (2) over 70,000 Brazilian transmigrants live in Germany, and many engage in Spiritist centers in major German cities; (3) I was able to detect direct Spiritist networks between Brazil and Germany; and (4) I was wondering how practices may resemble, differ, and transform between such different socio-cultural environments like Brazil and Germany. It was also a way to explore how it could be that I, as a German researcher, could become so much affected by local religious-spiritual practices in Brazil. I was curious if the mechanisms of sensory engagement I witnessed in Marília would work the same way in other environments in and outside Brazil. It was a way to compare Spiritist strategies of sensory manipulation in different interconnected care settings.

Hüwelmeier and Krause (2010) indicate that spirits travel with humans, and Bahia (2014) describes Brazilian religious practices in Germany as sites of identity (re)production in reference to Brazilian cultural symbols, permitting an individual expression of emotions and providing a sense of belonging in new contexts to relate and react to (ibid.: 358ff). These are aspects that appear highly relevant to me in terms of Transcultural Psychiatry, which relates the mental healthcare of migrants to their cultural idioms of distress, explanatory models, and socio-political implications (cf. Machleidt 2013). In this regard, new questions arise: Who communicates and contests Spiritist approaches to health in which way? How do people relate to Spiritism in different contexts? How do they frame, implement, and transform Spiritist practices and knowledge? And finally, what conflicts arise throughout processes of (local) implementation of Spiritist practices addressing health-related spiritual transformations?

The directory boards of the HEM ("Spiritist Hospital of Marília") and the CELV ("Spiritist Center of Light and Truth") in Marília highly estimate the communication, interaction, and reciprocity within a network of local, national, and global Spiritist institutions like the *Federaçao Espírita do Brasil* (FEB, "Spiritist Federation of Brazil"), the *Conselho Espírita Internacional* (CEI, "International Spiritist Council"), the *Associaçao Brasileira de Psicólogos Espírita* (ABRAPE, "Brazilian Association of Spiritist Psychologists"), and the *Associaçao Medico-Espírita* (AME, "Association of Spiritist Medicals") that each organize in regional, national, and international subgroups. These institutions provide spaces to meet Spiritists from other localities, establish cooperation and exchange programs for lecturers, discuss different perspectives on Spiritist knowledge and practice, and keep up with the newest interpretations and approaches. On some occasions, CAM are discussed, for example, Asian religious-spiritual models that focus on "frequencies and energetic forces channeled through our chakras" where, according to CELV's board member Taylor, spirits, and humans interact by "energetic vibration" to be dealt with in the context of mediumship and (dis)obsession (Interview 22 Nov. 2015). Maria-Helena, one of the mediumship trainees at HEM (and formerly CELV), pursues a similar approach and attracts members of the younger generation of Spiritists in Marília. She refers extensively to Dr. Alexandre, a health professional who tries to integrate biomedical, psychological, and spiritual knowledge. She complains that his attempts to establish projects regarding a "Spiritist medical science" are still being ignored by most of the "old-school" Spiritists who promote inner reform and study as proper methods. Juliana is one of her adepts who also engages with Dr. Alexandre, and I meet her in her merchandise shop in Marília. She is 34 years old and a single mother of 2. She tells me that she had to develop her mediumship out of emergency: she ran away from it all her life, having "weird experiences" and not knowing how to deal with them. Now, she would work as a medium to overcome her aversions "against society" by not only experiencing social support but also being able to help others. She admits that the study of Spiritist knowledge is essential to deal with cases of obsession and spiritual affliction but that it would be principally her weekly engagement with "energies" to balance herself and support others. She stresses the role of Dr. Alexandre as a medical doctor *and* Spiritist medium who academically engages with Spiritist healing practices.

Dr. Alexandre and Dr. Wilhelm

Dr. Alexandre performs within the *Centro Espírita Barsanulfo* (CEB, "Spiritist Center Barsanulfo"), which has existed since 1980 and was founded by former young adepts of CELV for the sake of implementing practice instead of just discussing it, as Juliana puts it (Interview 25 Jan. 2016). It is located between the economic center of Marília and its poorer suburbs. It offers free daycare for children to prevent them from loitering and running in the streets and to provide healthy nutrition in bodily and spiritual terms (e.g., learning about charity and solidarity in group activities and playful learning). The project is funded by the town administration of Marília, private donations, and a network of restaurant owners who support food supply with leftovers. A garden of self-grown vegetables and fruits complements nutrition and economic income, as does a small bookstore providing Spiritist literature. The vast territory also includes buildings for lectures, courses, mediumship sessions, and spiritual healing. Many young people of Marília's Spiritist community like to engage with Dr. Alexandre, who organizes courses on the interrelation of energetic healing ("psycho-physio-fluid-therapy") with somatic and psychological aspects of illness and health. He highlights concepts like chakras and energy fields deriving from oriental practices such as Reiki, Yoga, or Kundalini.

Every Monday night, Dr. Alexandre provides free "spiritual surgery" treatments in CEB. After I attended some of his classes, he invited me to participate in such a session in February 2016. He is a 44-year-old clinician and homeopath and turned to Spiritism at the age of sixteen, looking for rational explanations for spiritual experiences. He is part of the *Associaço Medico-Espírita* (AME, "Association of Spiritist Medicals") and has plans for a research project on the correlation of psycho-physio-fluid-therapy and cellular renewal but so far has lacked funding. Some of his assistants in the spiritual treatment are medical professionals and psychologists, too. Many also participate in his courses on Tuesdays, where they reflect on their experiences from the previous day and learn about the spiritual/energetic aspects of illness and health. Patients display a wide variety of chronic afflictions, but he only treats those who, according to him, suffer from spiritual/energetic issues. They usually receive at least a two-month treatment, which is structured in different episodes of consultation, mediumship sessions to explore spiritual aspects and to deal with cases of obsession, lectures, and an "extended *passe*," or, if indicated, "spiritual surgeries on the *perispirit*" of patients. After several weeks of participant observation, I deduced a few repetitive patterns of treatment, which I will summarize here in an idealized case format:

From 7 p.m. onward, people begin gathering in the Spiritist center's entrance area, chatting and having tea or water before entering a hall with eighty chairs, some marked with numbers. Some patients sit down right where they are; others receive a paper with a number and find their space in the rows of chairs, remaining quiet and trying to contemplate. In the background, meditative music is playing. An older man greets everyone personally and offers explanations and support for whoever is here for the first time. He tells them to relax, offers them something to read, and clarifies doubts about the procedure. He has been a patient himself and experienced support here; therefore, now he engages in supporting others. By 8 p.m., the room is packed with excited individuals chatting and discussing their situation until Dr. Alexandre enters a little stage in the front, turns off the music, and greets everybody. He says a prayer to ask for the guidance of God, Jesus, and "all the good spirits" before announcing that the lecture will be about different perspectives on "suffering." He summarizes his speech from the previous week on spiritual development and links it to today's subject by declaring that there are different forms of suffering: (1) limitation (to be surmounted by technology), (2) fear (to be overcome by knowledge), and (3) frustration (to be overcome by spiritual progress). Even though everybody would be free in their decision to progress, there would be "divine laws" framing this progression, including the "fact" that fraternity and charity serve the evolution of everybody and lead to satisfaction and happiness. Egoism and vanity, as provided by capitalism, would not support any progress but instead escalate in materialism and competition, leading to moral decline, violence, segregation, indifference, and, thus, to more suffering and expiration. In conclusion, humans create suffering through their improper acts and habits, but there will always be a chance for repentance and change: the study of Spiritist doctrine would help to progress and interrupt the vicious cycles of suffering. It includes that "sharing is caring" (see Chapter 3) and has more advantages than accumulating, thus providing hope, progress, and sustained healing as an act of self-transformation. He mentions that Pentecostals would still believe in magic, miracles, and salvation by external agencies instead of healing themselves, and this is why the knowledge of the causes of affliction and its spiritual aspects is of such importance. He continues with a "history of human suffering" that orients toward Xavier's *A Caminho Da Luz* (1939, "The Path of Light"), describing, analyzing, and interpreting examples of human suffering as related to historical epochal challenges and resolutions.

Apart from the structure of his argument, it is his performance as a speaker that affects me: his quite monotonous speech speeds up and slows down in rhythmic waves, taking me to another level of perception of "feeling" and "envisioning" what he refers to rather than cognitively processing it. At some point, I disconnect from the content of his lecture and feel taken by his voice and a sudden peaceful atmosphere in the room, as I did so often in similar environments (see Chapters 3 and 4). After his talk, Dr. Alexandre turns on the meditative music again and finishes with another prayer, thanking Jesus and the enlightened spirits for their support and the possibility of development and knowledge. Throughout his lecture of precisely one hour, participants have been called into another room to receive energetic treatment according to their numbers and remain to do so, while others are now standing around and chatting while waiting for the next phase of treatment: the "spiritual surgery" from 10 p.m. onward.

I have witnessed this practice several times, and on each occasion, it appeared to be different. Therefore, I will again exemplarily outline some structures and habits I regard as typical and add some individual case studies: In a room that is only illuminated by a single blue lightbulb on top of a desk, 15 participants of different ages and genders sit around 4 stretchers in a half-circle of chairs. Patients come in four by four after a woman at the desk reads their name, age, affliction, diagnosis, therapy aims, and progress. She defines the current treatment regulations, which usually consist of energetic manipulation of afflicted body parts by "mentalizing colors" and moving hands over the patients' bodies. She selects two persons to stand beside each stretcher. A person at the door calls in the patients who lay down on the stretchers, or in case it is too difficult for them, sit down in a chair. Meditative music plays in the background, and a person says a prayer, asking for spiritual support and "all the fluids and energies, belief and hope" they would need. The two persons on each stretcher perform an intensive *passe* on "their" patient. As indicated, it focuses on specific body parts and includes a "wiping off" toward their feet. Participants not actively involved in this practice are supposed to concentrate and "donate" energy until, after a few minutes, another thanksgiving prayer is performed, and the four patients are released by having a cup of "fluidized" water. Some even bring water bottles to take home as a daily remedy until they return the following week. Afterward, the person at the desk asks if anybody has made any specific observations, and related comments are added to the patient's file. Altogether, there are four rounds of ten minutes each, the last one also including participants. Regular issues are experiences of depression, anxiety, sadness, or emotional distress, but I also witness cases of sight loss, kidney stones, psychosis, auto-aggression, cancer, and auto-immune diseases. Dr. Alexandre explains to me that the treatment not only addresses certain body parts but also affects the chakras. At the intersection of Mesmerism and oriental practices, this energetic treatment aims at the dispersion of negative influences and the donation of positive energy waves called "fluids" as generated by the imagination of "colors." Patients are of different ages and genders, with a slight majority of middle-aged women. After the last patients leave the room, participants discuss involved spiritual aspects, addressing cases of obsession, karmic issues, and undeveloped mediumship. They agree on the necessity to guide these individuals toward Spiritist doctrine and practice and, in some instances, mediumship training. Some of their "insights" are based on psychographic messages produced in a room next door and constantly being handed to the therapists.

It took me some time to learn that as soon as Dr. Alexandre is engaged as a lecturer and/or healer, he serves as a medium for "spiritual healers" whom he "incorporates" and who allegedly talk and act through him. He declares that he is in contact with a spiritual team from a hospital in the spiritual sphere called *Esperança* ("hope") consisting of "strong spirits," most of them having been medical doctors or healers in one of their lifetimes. In the spiritual world, many spirits suffer from chronic issues to be resolved for spiritual progress, and, thus, they would decide to cooperate for reciprocal support: the "spirit doctors" help to treat the incarnate, and the mediums help to guide afflicted spirits toward realms of healing and progress (see Chapters 2 and 3). He would usually incorporate Dr. Wilhelm, a German medical doctor from Bavaria, who lived and practiced in World War I. Dr. Alexandre perceives it as a compelling and intense connection, as Dr. Wilhelm would "allow" him to stay conscious throughout the incorporation.[2] Together, they would intend to not only "energetically work on people" but also in psycho-therapeutic terms, for example, in the discussion of "spiritual messages." I was able to observe some cases on another occasion:

The procedure begins similarly to the before-mentioned ones, with the slight difference that there is only one stretcher in the center of the room. Around it, a circle of 12 chairs provides space for the participants, while another chair between the desk and the stretcher is reserved for Dr. Alexandre/Wilhelm. He sits there somewhat isolated, apparently highly concentrating and in a trance. The other participants gather in groups of 2 to 4, everyone silent. I learn that in contrast to the previous weeks, on this day, only two patients will be treated. The man at the desk invocates a prayer calling for the support of benevolent spirits and then discusses the case of the first patient who suffers from osteonecrosis in his femur. He then instructs three assistants to focus on the afflicted body parts and to "mentalize" specific colors in a fixed order. The patient enters, removes all metal devices that would "disturb energies," and lies on the stretcher. One medium positions at his head and invokes another prayer. Then, one after another, the three mediums perform their treatment on the left side of the patient while Dr. Alexandre/Wilhelm stays at his right side, observes, and only occasionally stretches out his hands as if to direct beams of energy. They move their hands over the patient's body in repeated movements. It looks like they remove specific energies and implement others. Dr. Wilhelm talks in a voice significantly different from Dr. Alexandre's regarding tone, speed, and accent. He also appears to embody different postures, performing significant and strange body habits like repeated shrugs and hand clasping. He "waves" from his belly toward the patient as if "donating energy" and then forms his hands in the shape of a tube and seems to blow and suck at the afflicted body part of the patient. He asks two other participants to help him and requests that the room be completely darkened. For a few minutes,

I can only hear murmurs. When the blue light is switched on again, all four have their hands placed on the right upper leg and hip of the patient. Dr. Wilhelm explains that they implanted a prosthesis in his *perispirit*. He asks the patient to cancel physiotherapy for the following two weeks so that it can heal. He also prescribes some homeopathic remedies and minerals, stressing that these suggestions derive from the spiritual world. After half an hour, the treatment finishes, and the second patient, who suffers from multiple sclerosis, enters the room. Again, the treatment begins with a similar procedure, just with the slight difference that throughout the initial prayer, she already receives energetic treatment by Dr. Alexandre/Wilhelm and his assistants in terms of "brushing away energies." They repeatedly rub their hands as if (dis)charging energies until she is instructed to turn around and, facing down, receives a massage by Dr. Alexandre/Wilhelm before turning back with an intense visible effort. Now, everybody in the room is asked to mentalize "green" and direct it to her whole body, particularly her lungs. Without any effort, I visualize a pair of lungs in front of my inner eye, which slowly transforms their diffuse appearance from a dirty see-through "color-lessness" to green and then to something I can, in synesthetic terms, best explain as a multisensory soothing experience of peace, harmony, and satisfaction. Dr. Alexandre/Wilhelm begins a conversation with the patient, declaring that there is a spirit around who allegedly had been her mother in an earlier incarnation, and that has obsessed her for the sake of resolving spiritual/karmic issues. For some time, I can barely hear what is said, but he is trying to persuade her that her illness is due to spiritual aspects such as karmic issues and amoral behavior. She cries a lot, posing one question after the other. Toward the end, I can understand better, and even though his voice is comforting, his message is not: he refers to his previous lectures and stresses that this case is about obsession and spiritual development. What shocks me most are his final words: she will not be healed in this life, but she has the chance to work on her spiritual progress to suffer less in her future lifetimes. Her affliction is auto-immune; her body does not accept the spirit, and, therefore, she would have to change her spiritual vibration. Having her obligatory cup of water, she leaves the room exclaiming excuses and sobbing. There is a long discussion about this case; finally, Dr. Alexandre/Wilhelm addresses me, pointing out how important my research would be and asking my opinion, but I can hardly pay any more attention; I leave the space with a hammering headache (Session 22 Feb. 2016).

Dr. Hermann

Dr. Hermann is another "German spirit doctor." He incorporates in his medium Paulo, who lives in Araraquara, about 230 km from Marília. He "works" in the local *Centro Espírita Casa do Caminho* (CECC, "Spiritist Center House of the Path") but also "tours" through the state of São Paulo and, thus, once a month comes to Marília. I first met him in February 2016 in Araraquara, but I learned about him from a member of the Spiritist community of Marília, Tatá, who is an author of Spiritist children's books and is currently compiling a historical account of HEM and Spiritism in Marília. I have never participated in any Spiritist practice with him, but he invited me several times to his house to talk about Spiritism in Marília. Tatá has been a Spiritist for over 30 years, and 10 years ago started to work with Paulo/Dr. Hermann. He would organize his monthly treatments at CELV until its administration decided not to support it anymore due to ideological considerations. Since then, he would organize it in the periphery of town. Tatá declares that Paulo has been seriously ill for years, suffering from diabetes and organic defects regarding his heart and lung functions, apart from being obese. He declares that many times, he feared that Paulo would not survive his exhausting therapeutic engagement. Being 58 years old, he would have already supported patients for more than 40 years. His altruistic behavior of attending anyone without limits or timetable would annoy many "more traditional" Spiritists who postulate a clear-cut delineated frame and structure of Spiritist healing practices. Tatá complains that these people acted just like political institutions aiming to control: to provide *passe*, you are required to attend a course on energetic healing and to support fellows in need of care spiritually, you must attend a course on Spiritist care and charity. He admits that knowledge is essential, but people forget about spontaneous "action in the name of love." He criticizes the prioritization of timetables and the fact that there are certain moments, hours, or days to heal instead of acknowledging "healing" as an everyday practice, obligation, and challenge.

Having Tatá's considerations in mind, I am still surprised to encounter Paulo as a *really* obese person. In his habitus, he appears quite the opposite of the straightforward Dr. Alexandre. In a slow and relaxed manner, Paulo shows me around his Spiritist center in Araraquara, starting with a second-hand shop where they sell donated clothes for an affordable price to gain some income for the center. Minutes later, I experience another surprise as Paulo guides me to his "pharmacy:" Apart from spiritually treating patients, he engages in phytotherapy and presents a massive storage of herbs, tinctures, and devices that remind me of a 19th-century drugstore. Glass bottles in all sizes, laboratory equipment, and staff in white coats who produce and mix remedies display a busy space of pharmaceutic fabrication and distribution. He states that this is all the work of Dr. Hermann, who instructs him and his assistants to gather over 150 different herbs "from the great pharmacy Brazil" and to prepare the remedies (Figures 5.1 and 5.2).

As in all Spiritist centers I have visited, treatment is free of charge, but donations are welcome. Patients arrive from 6 p.m. onward, receiving a paper with a number and writing their names in a book at the entrance. They stay waiting and relaxing, reading Spiritist literature until at 7 p.m., an

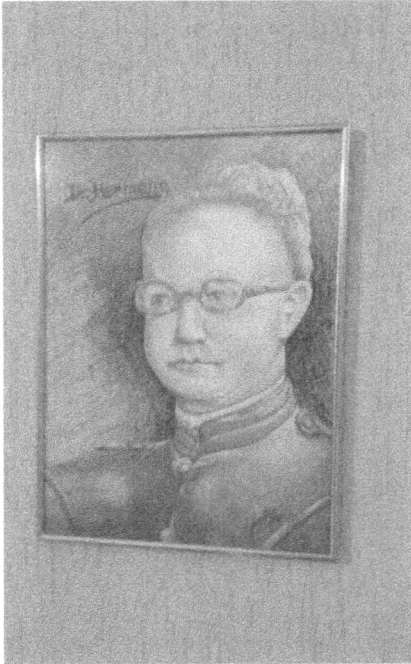

Figure 5.1 Psychographic Image of Dr. Hermann (Photography by HK 2016).

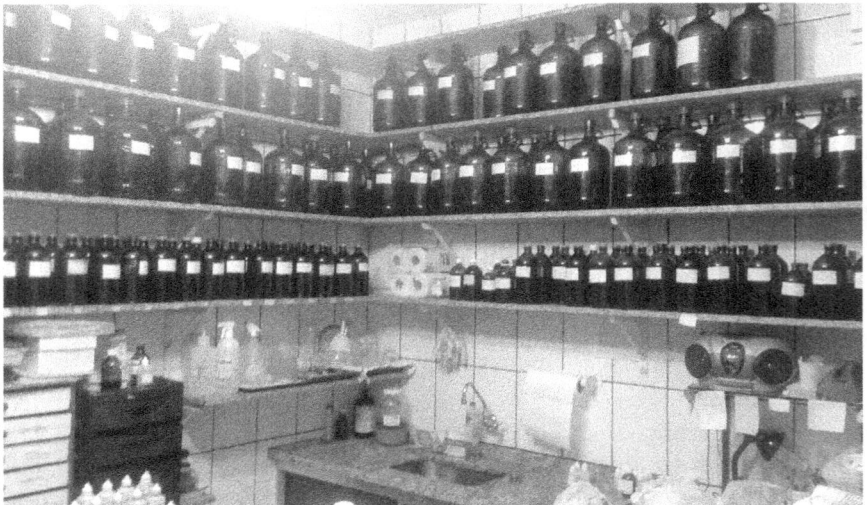

Figure 5.2 Dr. Hermann's Pharmacy (Photography by HK 2016).

assistant of Paulo enters a little stage, says a prayer, and discusses aspects of the Spiritist doctrine. In the smaller rooms, the therapeutic staff members prepare for the treatment: several mediums arrive that will incorporate members of Dr. Hermann's spiritual staff, which allegedly consists of 1300 entities who help him treat both patients and spirits. As in any hospital, patients suffer from various afflictions as, according to Paulo, any somatic problem would have spiritual aspects and vice versa. However, most would suffer from nervousness, anxiety, stress, or sadness. The treatment would usually affect the body through the remedies, the *perispirit* through energetic treatment, and the spirit through the spiritual transformation with lectures, studies, and the adaption to a Spiritist lifestyle. The treatment room resembles a medical doctor's office with a huge desk, piles of patients' files, some requisites that look like medical instruments, and various bottles with liquids. A stretcher is at the center of the room, with several chairs around it. The air is soaked by a fresh fragrance made of avocado seeds, but it reminds me of disinfectant.

By 9 p.m., ten persons (Paulo, three other men, and six women) gather in the treatment room lit only by a blue lightbulb. Some wear white coats, and throughout the session, the number of persons changes as some leave the room and others enter. Paulo/Dr. Hermann sits down behind the desk in silence and says a prayer in a different voice that sounds rougher but more jovial. He now speaks with a strong accent and greets me as his "German fellow." Then he goes from one person to another, shaping his hands like a bowl and allegedly taking out bad energies, which he "places" in a corner of the room. He sits down again and skips through the patients' files, giving instructions and prescribing remedies, their composition, and modes of application according to the information he finds. A staff member writes everything down and hands the notes to a colleague who leaves for the "pharmacy" to prepare everything. Patients enter through a door from the waiting area, and Paulo/Dr. Hermann interviews them on their condition. He provides further treatment instructions written down in the patient's file and, in some cases, performs an energetic treatment comparable to his initial practice. In other cases, he uses the spray of avocado seeds and applies it to afflicted body parts by rubbing it in and then cleaning it with a paper towel. In between, a medium transmits messages on spiritual or karmic issues of specific patients, and Paulo/Dr. Hermann comments on the patient's behavior or spiritual development. After 10–20 minutes, patients leave the room through another door toward the "pharmacy" to receive their remedies and written instructions. By 1 a.m., the last patient leaves, and after some explanations and instructions to the staff, Paulo/Dr. Hermann finishes the session with another prayer.

The following day, I meet Paulo and his wife at their nearby home within the same middle-class residential area. He shares his life story with me that resembles the narratives of other mediums I have met before (see Chapters 3 and 4): from the age of approximately six years old, he started to see spirits that his Catholic priest identified as "demons." He provided no further explanation or support but advice to pray. Later, Paulo began to frequent a Spiritist center, and from eighteen years onward, he engaged in mediumship practices to find the right way to deal with these experiences. He would now identify it as a gift of God to receive the possibility of resolving karmic debts, but back then, he rejected Dr. Hermann as a fruit of his imagination, something wanting to drive him crazy. Still, it was there and insisted, and there are parts of his life that it helped him a lot with. Even though he experiences it as a difficult task to collect all the herbs and provide treatment at least once a week, he also experiences "peace of spirit/mind," sleeps better, and gets along with other people more easily. Before, he would have to take tranquilizers that a psychiatrist had prescribed to him, but which would only make things worse. Now, he would follow his intuition not only for his life decisions but also regarding the plants, remedies, and the treatment of people. He declares that patients would seek Dr. Hermann's support usually only after they did not experience any support or therapy success with "terrestrial doctors" or religious institutions. Often, people would experience discrimination due to their symptoms and/or financial status and would not have access to proper therapy facilities. He would, thus, also serve to cushion the health-political maldevelopments in Brazil (Interview 12 Feb. 2016).

As mentioned before, Paulo/Dr. Hermann regularly travels the state of São Paulo and, once a month, stays for a weekend in Marília and treats patients from Saturday morning until late at night. Having been abandoned by CELV, the sessions now occur in a small Spiritist center within a *favela*. The entire day, volunteers from the Spiritist community of Marília (including HEM and CELV but with a higher age average than from CEB) organize lectures, prayer groups, live music with spiritual contents, a bazaar for affordable second-hand or home-made items, and free meals for everybody. Patients come with all kinds of afflictions and are suffering from more impoverished living conditions than it seems to be at CEB. The context resembles more the observations and experiences I made in the Northeastern state of Bahia than any other experience in the Southeastern state of São Paulo regarding relative poverty and the quality of (healthcare) infrastructures.

Dr. Claudionor

Itabuna resembles Marília in size and function as a local center of commerce and administration, but due to relative poverty, it lacks infrastructure maintenance. Whereas Marília only bears "problematic neighborhoods" at its margins, Itabuna provides very few wealthy quarters, and if so, they are fenced off with barbed and electric wires. Lifestyle is rustic, but strangers in the street are as friendly and open-minded to foreigners even though, or maybe because, they are rare here. Tourists usually only stay a few hours to move on to the beach resorts of Itacaré, about 100 km away, or to change buses to other destinations. It takes me as a surprise that at the several Spiritist centers of town – in relative comparison to Marília, half the concentration in spatial and population terms – I am received with awe and that it takes weeks to establish some careful trust with a few members of the *Centro Espírita Claudionor de Carvalho* (CECC, "Spiritist Center of Claudionor de Carvalho"). It may be because, within a more impoverished and mainly Afro-Brazilian community, the *gringo* appears out of place or is deemed a curious tourist who wants to witness some "exotic practice." However, with time, I learn that people are cautious toward any stranger who asks too many questions due to hostile and competitive behaviors from Evangelical/Pentecostal actors in their direct vicinity.

CECC is located at the periphery of Itabuna, on the outskirts of the suburb of Santo Antonio, with its dirt roads full of stray dogs, human and animal excrement, homeless people, criminals, drug dealers, and unregistered businesses. In a building that resembles a renovated former industrial complex, the spirit of deceased medical doctor Claudionor de Carvalho engages in healing (Figure 5.3). He allegedly lived and practiced a century ago in the state of São Paulo and now incorporates twice a week in his medium Marcus to treat patients, specializing in symptoms of depression

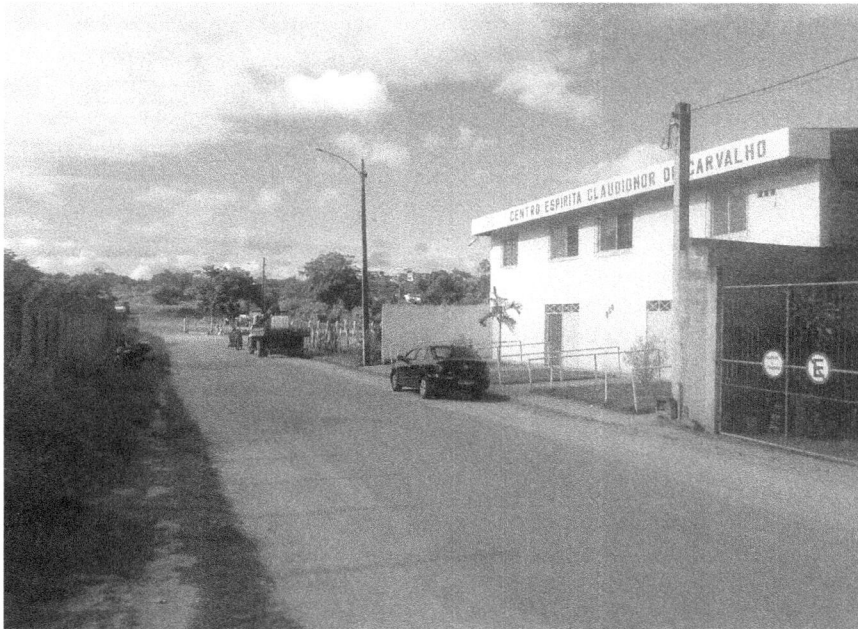

Figure 5.3 Front view of the *Centro Espírita Claudionor de Carvalho* (Photography by HK 2016).

and cardiovascular problems. He offers complementary therapy to biomedical approaches and demands that patients participate at least once a week in a lecture and follow certain dietary, sexual, and behavioral restrictions according to their energetic state. Treatment continues for at least eight weeks but sometimes even for years and, just as in Marília, consists of study, disobsession, and energetic therapy. It is free of charge, but donations are readily accepted. Other acts of charity are performed on Wednesdays when inhabitants of the relatively poor neighborhood come to listen to spiritual lectures and receive free soup, while social workers and other volunteers attend their children to discuss life issues and problems in school and spend the afternoon in a friendly and relaxing atmosphere. Families whose members come every week receive donated staple foods once a month.

CECC members also organize non-spiritual medical treatment arranged by volunteer Renata. She is 35 years old, unmarried, and the mother of a 5-year-old daughter. She works as a nurse at the public hospital of Itabuna and has a master's degree in public healthcare. She criticizes the conditions of the Brazilian healthcare system and "her" hospital in particular: "It used to be a great hospital, where everyone was attended, but due to recent health policy, now it is on the level of cavemen" (Interview 17 Feb. 2017). Renata relates to herself as a medium, and throughout her entire life, she has attended sessions in various Spiritist centers, also because of her Spiritist mother. A few years ago, she stopped working as a medium due to her exhaustion from work and the education of her daughter. It was when, in her terms, she started to feel that she was becoming "crazy." She mentions diagnoses of depression and anxiety, which she initially had treated by a psychiatrist but then decided to see Dr. Claudionor. He diagnosed that her affliction was related to her undeveloped mediumship, allowing spirit obsessors to energetically harm her *perispirit* and, thus, her body and mind. For many months, he and his helping team, including psychologists, physiotherapists, teachers, and former patients, took care of her. She attended study groups and lectures and slowly started to work as a medium again, providing peace of mind to her and having her engage in disobsession again. Furthermore, Renata began to establish the project "Francis of Assisi," a family health endeavor taking care of children from the problematic *favela* environment. She and other Spiritist volunteers visit families' homes and provide psycho-social support regarding family conflicts. With her nursery skills, she also distributes first aid and amnesic for people in need, whom she then passes on to a network of medical doctors who treat people free of charge, apart from the public health system, which often implies long commutes, extended waiting, and marginal treatment. One of these medicals, a Spiritist herself, even visits CECC once a week to provide free diagnosis and medication. As mentioned before, unlike Marília, Itabuna offers marginal living standards to most of its inhabitants, including a high rate of unemployment and restricted access to healthcare.

CECC thus does not address patients so much in terms of complementary treatment but even more as a substitute for the marginal public healthcare system. However, there is Healing Cooperation in the sense that spiritual and academically trained health professionals support each other even in referring patients from "conventional" to "spiritual" treatment and vice versa. Spiritual treatment at CECC is structured as follows:

On Mondays, Marcus/Dr. Claudionor consults patients and decides if they need spiritual treatment. His focus is on cases of depression and related symptoms. Those diagnosed with spiritual problems will receive energetic therapy in terms of an elaborated form of *passe* focusing on the patient's chakras by about twenty assistants, in many aspects analogous to practices at CEB in Marília. CECC resembles a private clinic with a waiting area where people read or listen to Spiritist doctrine, examination rooms and offices, and a therapy room with six stretchers where patients lay down to receive energetic treatment in a quiet atmosphere with a darkened, greenish light and mellow music in the background (Figure 5.4). Information on any patient is logged in personalized files, and they are supposed to write a diary where they report their daily routines and spiritual progress. Based on these files and reports, Marcus/Dr. Claudionor provides instructions for future treatment. On Tuesdays, he receives patients with cardiovascular and related

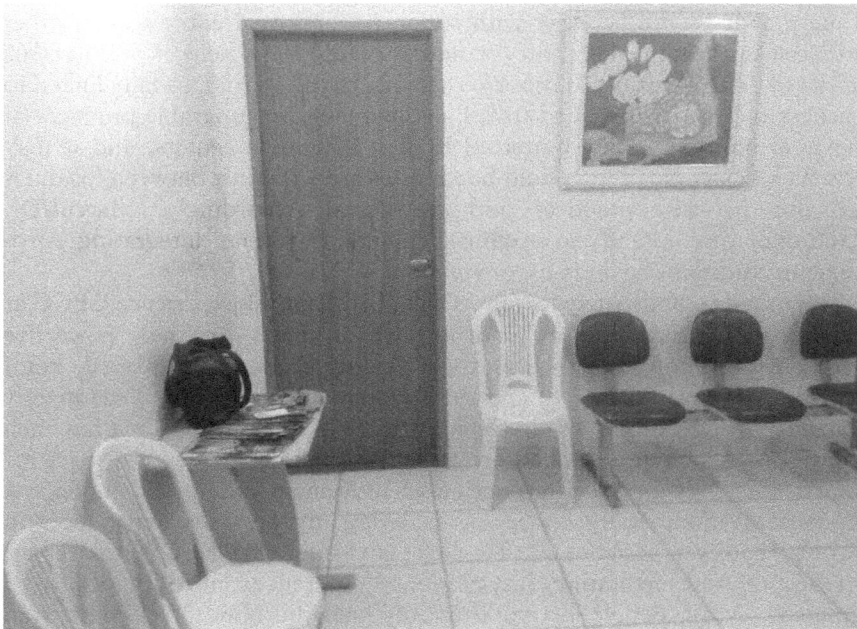

Figure 5.4 CECC's Waiting Room (Photography by HK 2016).

problems and actively participates in the treatment, going from stretcher to stretcher, checking the condition of the patients, and performing "spiritual surgeries" by applying different wadding with liquids and band-aids. Afterward, his assistants will perform chakra treatment like on Mondays, according to a detailed application manual. When Marcus/Dr. Claudionor diagnoses influences of obsessing spirits, they are addressed in disobsession meetings on Thursdays. A group of mediums and assistants meet for several hours, and the procedure is structured as follows: three persons will sit together: a medium, an instructor, and a secretary. The secretary reads out the case from the patient's file, and immediately, the medium receives the obsessing spirit and reveals its motives. The instructor will then get into a conversation with the spirit, trying to receive more information and to convince the spirit of its wrong behavior, and, in the best case, having it pass on to the spiritual plane, where it will receive further guidance by supporting spirits (see Chapter 3). The secretary notes every detail in the patients' files so Dr. Claudionor can later decide about future steps. His medium, Marcus, suffers from ill health himself, but I was never able to discuss it as he would only reveal himself to me as Dr. Claudionor, apart from one conversation I had with him in 2011, still exploring "my field." On one occasion that I participated in his treatments, he stressed that this was a clinic and not a religious site and that many medical doctors would send their chronic patients here when their treatment lacked therapy success. He also explained to me that he is not as strict with supportive spiritual entities as in other Kardecist institutions: here, they would also accept the help of *preto velhos* (spirits of "old slaves") and *caboclos* ("Indigenous" spirits), usually linked to practices of *Umbanda*. Vice versa, I also witnessed comparable practices of "hospital mimicry" (cf. Montero 1985) in *Umbanda* centers, and it may serve as an example of how fluid boundaries are – not just between localities but also between practices and ideologies. Accordingly, Marcus/Dr. Claudionor also intends to establish community events integrating Afro-Brazilian traditions such as *capoeira*.

Compared to Spiritist spaces in Marília/São Paulo, I experience CECC as less organized and "louder," but it also accounts for their respective environment. Upon arrival, music with spiritual content is played, but I perceive it as less meditative, and the speakers are screeching. I see mainly women chatting as their children play with each other and only a few men who sit down in the quieter corners of the vast hall that serves as a space for lectures and study groups. The continuous movement and noise do not allow for concentration, at least when considering my previous experiences in Marília. However, compared to the direct environment, CECC is still a space of reflection and meditation, just gradually different from other localities I witnessed. Most people derive from the neighborhood, but some staff members, lecturers, and volunteers, who not only sacrifice their leisure time here to support others but also accept long traveling hours, come from other parts of town or the region. One of them is Maria, a 44-year-old teacher who has been interested in Spiritism before but only has engaged at CECC since 2004 after experiencing healing herself:

> I had this terrible pain in my arm that even kept me from sleeping. I went to the doctor and underwent some diagnostics, but no therapy would succeed. So, I came to the fraternal care and passed *fluidoterapia* and disobsession, as back in the day, the patient would still participate. The communication was unbelievable and helped me a lot. Gradually, I frequented more, helping distribute, writing things down during disobsession, and participating in the study. And then Marcus would teach about this whole chakra thing, and the therapy was done, and I would not feel anything anymore. So, I started to participate more and more in therapy. Moreover, I had terrible eating behavior, not eating properly until Dr. Claudionor told me one day during the treatment of a client that I would have stomach problems because I would eat shit, whereas this patient would probably die of hunger. That was a turning point, and I started to eat healthier, also to be able to help others more profoundly.
>
> (Interview 21 Jan. 2017)

It is evident that these narratives, as well as those presented in the previous subchapters, in one way or another, align personal experiences and practices to local frameworks that evolve from broader socio-cultural, political, and economic conditions in Brazil. This context raises the question of how they might apply to other parts of the world. Once we already know that they do so, I intend to explore further how they are implemented and transformed to adapt to divergent local frames outside Brazil, particularly Germany, as one of the breeding grounds of Spiritism about two centuries ago (see Chapter 2).

Spiritism 2.0 in Germany

Apart from Brazil, Spiritism also contributes its healing practices to a growing landscape of CAM (cf. Ross 2012) in other countries, including North America and Europe (Lewgoy 2008). As indicated in Chapter 2, US-American psychologist Bragdon engages in implementing Spiritist practices into her program of Integrative Mental Health as a combination of evidence-based and alternative therapy methods (Bragdon 2012a). Another example of the transnational distribution of Brazilian Spiritism is the before-mentioned John of God (see Chapter 2; cf. Rocha 2017), who mainly attracts chronic patients from all over the world to his Spiritist center in Abadiana/Minas Gerais/Brazil. To promote his spiritual healing practices, he also travels the world, including Germany and other European destinations (cf. Voss 2011: 31f, 226f).

Whereas investigative approaches focusing on the implementation of spiritual practices as CAM in "Western" contexts highlight conceptional intersections and fusions with New Age practices and dissolution from ethnic, religious, or national characterized clienteles (cf. Heelas 2011; Baer et al. 2013), migration-related research provides contradictory data: it displays a more diversified heterogeneity regarding the adaption and implementation of Spiritist practices. It is especially true for the Spiritist branch of *Umbanda*, which, in different European settings such as England (cf. Sterzi 2011) or Portugal (cf. Saraiva 2010), displays opposing diasporic identity formation patterns. They offer coping strategies for alienation, homesickness, identity loss, and depression in a homogeneous cultural and linguistic environment apart from spaces of transcultural communication, integration, and mutual support in times of critical emotional affliction and experiences.

Various researchers have addressed facets of Brazilian transmigration to different countries and their respective strategies of interaction, adaption, and negotiation of "identity," but almost none of these contributions have focused on religious-spiritual and health-related aspects. However, Messias (2002) acknowledges that in taking care of their health, Brazilian migrants often rely on a combination of personal and collective transnational resources. They would move back and forth across informal and formal healthcare systems, crossing multiple national, cultural, and healthcare system borders. Accordingly, Brazilian migrants in Germany also implement Spiritist well-being and (self-)care practices. Since the 1990s, Brazilian communities have established Spiritist centers in major German cities, most associated with the *Deutsche Spiritistische Vereinigung* (DSV, "German Spiritist Association"). DSV is directly connected to FEB through the Brazilian-dominated CEI and invites lecturers to Germany, including Divaldo Franco (see Chapter 2) and Andrei Moreira (see Chapter 1), promoting health and spiritual well-being in line with Spiritism. Members of AME travel to Europe, particularly Germany, discussing therapeutic-spiritual aspects with Brazilian immigrants and German adepts. Particularly, the latter have recently engaged in discussing the implementation of Spiritist explanatory models and therapeutic practices into the German health system. One of the more prominent examples is the organizer of the annual *PsychoMedizin Kongress* in Bad Honnef (see Chapter 2), who invites Brazilian Spiritists to share their knowledge with a wide range of "alternative" therapists and an interested public. When I participated in 2016, two aspects irritated me: first, many participants were not capable of understanding Spiritist approaches due to socio-cultural differences in concepts of self, person, and explanatory models regarding health and illness, and second, the immense participation fee contradicted the charitable approach of Spiritists in Brazil. To my knowledge, this has not changed until today and might mark an adaption to the German environment where some clientele expect to pay a high price for sustained treatment that is not readily available to everyone.

In contrast, DSV aspires to implant solidarity and fraternal care by providing and coordinating Spiritist practice in Germany. In 2016, I participated in their annual meeting in Frankfurt/Main, which took the form of a scientific congress with keynotes, presentations, lectures, workshops, and book tables. At first sight, the meeting seemed to serve the exchange between Brazilian communities in Germany, and one contested topic was the role of the German language in Spiritist centers: some argued that Spiritist centers should be a refuge for Brazilian immigrants and the maintenance of their cultural identity, whereas others saw them as a space of integration, exchange, and the elaboration of the Spiritist doctrine in Germany. The latter's central argument would be that Spiritism is not to be understood as a Brazilian cultural practice but as a universally valid and scientifically elaborated way of life that has only been preserved in Brazil until it could be globally distributed again (cf. Xavier 1938; see Chapter 2). Accordingly, Spiritism would have to deny its religious-cultural implication to be accessible to people worldwide.

DSV members emphasized three central practices that closely copy the Brazilian model: the study of Spiritist doctrine, spiritual assistance, and mediumship training. The study would be necessary for the individual to develop a Spiritist habitus summarized in the following six aspects: learning, reflection, internalization, experiences of change, transformation, and being an example for others. It would also require assisting others spiritually and offering moral support to those in need, following the example of Jesus Christ. This attitude implies welcoming others open-mindedly and offering empathetic fraternal care, lectures to "touch people's hearts," and joint prayers. The energetic treatment (*passe*) would be central, too – not as a medical treatment but as a technique to calm down and connect with clients. Mediumship would be a practice that includes study, integration, respect, discipline, and love. It has been defined as a natural sensation of spiritual influences, which means that every human being can sense spirits, and individual differences originate from the respective sensory organization of the body. To practice mediumship, adepts would need sustained skills to differentiate internal and external sources of sensation. They would have to focus their attention on sensory details, using certain practices and techniques: silence and relaxation would be the necessary conditions for any spiritual communication and would enable spirits to establish contact. Accordingly, the recollection of mind and self allows mediums to be at ease with themselves and thus to interact with spirits and others. Techniques for ridding disturbing thoughts include prayer and reading, as well as oriental meditation practices that would help to focus on the attention to others and personal aims. Alertness is promoted as a core of mediumship: thoughts and emotions should not be suppressed but controlled. Internal reform and study would change modes of perception, vibration, and energetic states and support a sustained inner reform in terms of self-transformation and the capacity to help others.

It is obvious how these guidelines discussed within the DSV meeting in 2016 correspond to my analysis of Spiritist healing practices in Brazil (see Chapters 3 and 4). However, in Brazil, they have never been outlined so clear-cut, not even by the most influential authors of Spiritist literature (see Chapter 2). It is a synthesis of my observations and experiences as a German after years of field research in Brazil, which is now in such a casual manner shared here. I am convinced it is another adaptation to the German environment to explain aspects of Spiritist practice in such a structured way. I decided to explore further how Spiritist practice and knowledge are implemented in Spiritist centers in Germany in sensory and embodied terms. Again, I followed connections within a translocal network, which in this case were initiated by Maria-Helena (see Chapter 4) and her daughter, who lives in Munich, Germany. She is affiliated with a Spiritist center there and has facilitated my access.

In 2016 and 2017, I conducted participant observation and narrative interviews within the Spiritist center *Grupo Espírita de Estudos Allan Kardec* (GEEAK; "Spiritist Study Group of Allan Kardec") in Munich. I observed contradicting and contested approaches and positions regarding integrating Spiritism into the German healthcare system that would eventually induce the group's separation. It was established in the early 1990s by Brazilian immigrants and has aimed at providing and promoting Spiritist practice through charity, prayer, and the study of the Spiritist doctrine, according to Allan Kardec. Fifty to sixty members regularly participate in lectures, study groups, and fluidic treatment (*passe*), and around ten persons engage in a mediumship training course. Twenty percent are Germans, while the other eighty percent comprises persons of Brazilian descent. Once a week, a study group of 10–15 participants discusses Spiritist literature in the German language in a round-table manner: one after another, participants read aloud a paragraph and discuss how it would apply to their experiences. Unlike this, on another day, a Portuguese-speaking group assembles to listen to lectures of GEEAK volunteers or guests from other Spiritist centers in Brazil or Germany who discuss certain aspects of life from the perspective of Spiritism.[3] The aesthetic framing with meditative music, prayers, dimmed light, and performance of *passe* in both settings resembles many of my experiences in Brazil elaborated above, but it becomes apparent that the "German group," including Brazilians that already have lived in Germany for many years, promotes more active engagement with discussions on the doctrine than the relatively passive "Brazilian group" does. Whereas the former discusses specific aspects of the literature, the latter prefers to relate it to daily issues within a peer group of similar socio-cultural Brazilian descent. Apart from a few individuals who like to participate in both groups for integration, interaction, and communication, most members remain dedicated to only one of these groups. This dynamic is intensified by a shared practice of prejudice and mutual rejection in which some Brazilians assume that Germans are not capable of fully understanding the Spiritist doctrine due to a lack of knowledge and empathetic skills, whereas some German members complain about the arrogance, organizational failures, and lack of alleged basic structures in the implementation of Spritist practice and knowledge within the German context.

This contest, which, regarding my observations in Chapters 3 and 4, appears contrary to the Spiritist ideology of solidarity and charity, becomes most apparent when addressing mediumship training and practice. For years, a relatively small group of Brazilian participants has engaged in weekly mediumship training and disobsession practices. Recently, the group also has started to accept German participants, but discussions on language evolved, which is why they have split into two groups, quarreling about "correct" approaches such as if German spirits' messages should be transmitted in German or Portuguese language. Furthermore, all members of this officially charitable association pay small monthly contributions according to their capabilities, and sometimes bazaars are organized to gather more income. In particular, the Brazilian part of the group regularly celebrates birthday parties and other social events in "a Brazilian way," where most German members rarely are invited to participate. Accordingly, apart from a few Brazilians who engage in both, the two groups rarely interact because German members, most of them not being partners of Brazilian members, come for spiritual engagement devoid of national or cultural denomination.

Mike, for example, is a 49-year-old German who has worked as a courier for 18 years. He is unmarried, childless, and only has a few family ties in another German region. He appears to have few social contacts but has a strong will to compensate for it with altruistic behavior. He has participated in the Spiritist center for seven years, ever since he suffered "blackouts" which had never been clinically diagnosed. He had contacts with Brazilians at that time, and since he mentioned once, during his blackouts, that he would feel the presence of somebody, one of them suggested that he might be a medium and took him to the center. His medical doctor concluded that he suffered from stress and dehydration, but by then, he was already attuned to the center and impressed by the "open-hearted attitude" of people who would accept him "like a brother." He soon felt that the Spiritist doctrine was something he was always convinced of but could not grasp. He wanted to participate in the mediumship training group right away but had to accept that he was deemed to be not prepared enough and would have to study first. It would not work in linguistic terms either, as the studies were conducted in German but with mediumistic messages in Portuguese. Still, he felt that now he could develop spiritually and had finally "arrived home." He perceives the group as the extended family he never had and, for the first time in his life, has felt entirely accepted. He does not experience it as a form of healing, but it helps him to take better care of himself; he declares that he needs "soul food," a path to follow, and an aim. He started to learn how to perform *passe* three or four years ago, and for two years now, he has participated in the mediumship group. However, he does not perceive himself as a "classical medium" that listens to voices or sees spirits but as intuitive, empathetic:

> The most beautiful thing is to help, to practice charity. And if it is not for a living person, I do it for the spiritual world. [...] You feel this satisfaction, this happiness, and I sometimes cry with bliss. Knowledge is important, but without practice, it does not value anything. There is no use in accumulating knowledge your whole life if you cannot put it into practice. When I die, nobody will ask me how many books I have read, but what I have done. We had so many discussions over here about how to practice charity, but this is obsolete. You must do what you think is right and follow your gut. Rational thinking is not always helpful.
>
> (Interview 21 Sep. 2016)

From this quote, it becomes apparent that Mike has embodied Spiritist knowledge and how his access and experience resemble the narratives of many Brazilian Spiritists (see Chapters 3 and 4). However, he does not perceive Spiritist practices as healing techniques but as a support of well-being, which he defines as a symbiosis of care and self-care. He acknowledges Brazil's importance in the development of Spiritism but does not hold it as a Brazilian socio-cultural practice: the fusion of ethnicities is the base for global Spiritist knowledge, and now, it is redistributed to the world again. When this task is accomplished, Brazil will not hold any particular position anymore; they did their job to preserve the doctrine – not more, not less (ibid.).

Heike is a 55-year-old German unmarried woman who works in the service unit of a public transportation company. She perceives herself as a medium and describes her mediumship as an inner voice that, since the age of six, has warned her of dangerous situations and helped her with daily decisions. She believes she can travel to the spiritual world in her dreams and communicate with the spirits of deceased persons. She has been reading literature on mediumship and New Age spirituality all her life and came to GEEAK more by accident, researching for additional information online. It would help her to talk to people who share, understand, and appreciate her experience and to develop her knowledge with the lectures and study groups. She has participated in GEEAK since 2012, a time that she describes as very sorrowful: within a few years, she lost her parents, a friend, and a colleague she liked a lot. Other unlucky events and difficult experiences have added up and left her desperate. When she became a member of GEEAK, she enjoyed the attention and empathy of this new peer group. Heike believes that it was her misfortune that brought her here and that God gave her all these issues to resolve and spiritually develop. She perceives the studies and discussions as a regeneration of her inner self, which also helps her to deal with difficult life situations and avoid stress. She participates in the mediumship training group, claiming that this is what she always wanted: having the possibility to help afflicted spirits and releasing negative energies and influences, which she would accumulate in her daily life. To her, it is her vocation, and she is happy that she can realize it within this community:

> I am here to carry out my obligations, and this mediumship has not been given to me for nothing. It feels right, and there must be people to increase the vibration of this planet. For this, we have to deal with spiritual beings, and there are not enough people doing so. I feel that this is right.
>
> (Interview 13 Jun. 2017)

Accordingly, Heike integrates Spiritist knowledge and practice as an explanatory model for experiences she has had her whole life and as a way to not only cope with them but also to fold them into her daily practice. However, Heike, just like Mike, is one of the members of GEEAK who will split and establish a new group. It leaves her very sad but is necessary due to the contrary expectations and aims of members and participants. In her opinion, many Brazilians would create "their little nest to hide in," while other members are more ambitious regarding the implementation of Kardecist doctrine into German health discourse and practice. She considers it a cultural problem and criticizes the approach of Brazilian Spiritists who only talk about God, Jesus, and Kardec. There are many possible paths, and she wants to do what feels good and right. Like Mike, she does not perceive it as therapy, but it helps her be more attentive to herself and reflect on the causes and effects of personal problems. Her narrative resembles many examples of my Brazilian research partners who have engaged in Spiritism to cope with lifelong deviant (mediumistic?) experiences. On the contrary, many Brazilians at GEEAK only started to engage with Spiritism after arriving in Germany, like, for example, Fernanda.

Fernanda is from the city of São Paulo, 32 years old, and she studied industrial design in Brazil. Born into a Catholic family, ever since adolescence, she has developed an atheist and antireligious worldview. In 2009, at the age of 25, she entered Germany with a student visa to study the German language and culture. She never attended university classes but instead has tried to work in her profession. As her Brazilian academic graduation was not accepted in Germany, she started to feel exploited in low-wage internships, a fact that humiliated and frustrated her, and finally developed into a clinical depression. According to her, this was when she began engaging with God again because she had been suffering so much and needed something to hold on to and to support her. In 2013, she met her future German husband, Peter, who has emotionally supported her and warrants her legal status in Germany. From 2014 on, she has frequented GEEAK and actively participates in both the Brazilian and German lectures and study groups, convincing her husband to accompany her in the latter. To Fernanda, participation within GEEAK has been crucial to getting back on track since she no longer knew how to deal with her situation as a skillful and ambitious young woman who, with her immigrant status, became marginalized in German society. Presently, it is essential to her to support others who are having comparable experiences, and she believes that GEEAK provides possibilities to do so:

> Since I have been here, I experienced inner reform. I have been working on my inner self by reading and lectures. I learned a lot, and I think that it helped me to initiate major changes. Back in the day, I was lofty and full of mistakes, but here, I have worked it out to be humble. I learned it with Spiritism. [...] It was a relief to work on myself because I saw that the world would not change that easy – so I have to change my perspective on the world.
>
> (Interview 28 Sep. 2016)

Fernanda is convinced that the Spiritist practice and community helped her overcome her problems in finding coping strategies and new perspectives in life. She tells me about past periods of severe depression and suicidal tendencies, but I experience her as a woman who has been able to transgress disturbing experiences and develop agency in a hostile environment toward migrants due to the spiritual support of fellow GEEAK members. Now, she is an independent, self-employed graphic designer and enjoys interacting with both the Brazilian and German groups in GEEAK. She is shocked and sad when she learns that the group will split in 2017 and finally renounces herself from any Spiritist activities. Since then, she seems to engage more with oriental impressions of spirituality and mindfulness that she loves to share with others through social media. Fernanda's example supports my argument that cultural aspects of a peer group are of specific importance, but personal expectations, individual resources, and political contexts are central to the translocal distribution of models of healing and well-being. Both Fernanda and Heike refer to GEEAK as a place of well-being in a difficult life situation, but their narratives differ regarding personal experiences. Fernanda suffers from a hostile political context regarding the integration of immigrants and develops a clinical depression with suicidal tendencies. She declares that it was only through this support group and their reference to Brazilian solidarity practices that she could recover – although Spiritism has not been her life orientation before. At the same time, participation in the German study group helps her to integrate into the new cultural context, which is why she is disappointed about its loss by separation. Over the years, she has learned to highly estimate GEEAK as a transitional space where she could connect her Brazilian background to her life reality in Germany. In contrast, Heike has had spiritual experiences that she cannot communicate to others without the danger of being labeled as *verrückt* ("crazy"), seeking shelter where she can express her experiences. However, like many other long-term Brazilian and German members, she is annoyed by the impact of Brazilian (religious) cultural aspects and wants to adjust Spiritist practice to the German context, customs, and requirements.

The different narratives of Fernanda, Heike, and Mike reflect patterns of distinctive pathways to Spiritism in Brazil and Germany. My observations support the idea that Brazilian migrants, who have not been Spiritists before, experience the Spiritist center more as a place of well-being (cf. Ferraro & Barletti 2016) where they can reflect on and handle their daily experiences in a foreign country within a "Brazilian environment." To a certain degree, the German members understand that their Brazilian fellows have suffered from structural violence and seek relief in an environment that provides a protecting "nest" of Brazilian cultural belonging *and*, at the same time, a more challenging mixed German-Brazilian environment of integration. However, conflicts are emerging, starting with German and "progressive" Brazilian members of GEEAK no longer agreeing on the Portuguese language used in mediumship practices and other contexts. As my last case study of Sandra will illustrate in an instance, many entities incorporated in the mediums were "German" spirits, so participants wondered why they would communicate in Portuguese. Some argued that to share feelings and sensations, a medium should communicate their experiences in a language they are comfortable with, but at GEEAK, this question became a political issue of identity, belonging, and adaptation to socio-cultural frames and contexts.

Sandra is a Brazilian mother of two and divorced from her German husband. She organizes another Spiritist practice – the Gospels at Home (see Chapter 4) – visiting affiliated but immobile persons in Munich and the neighboring towns. Volunteers would provide this service twice a week for persons who cannot visit GEEAK due to illness or infrastructural problems. As her counterpart Renata at CECC in Itabuna, her aim is not to proselytize but to offer psycho-social and spiritual support to people in need. Sandra tells her story as a coherent narrative where one incident has led to the other in Spiritist terms: she has had mediumship experiences since the age of eight years, and her father, an herbalist, ensured that she would protect herself by studying Spiritist literature. Twenty years ago, she came to Germany with her boyfriend, and it was a turning point in her life: she perceived that she had lived in Germany before and recognized the parents of her boyfriend as her former parents. She confesses that in this former lifetime, she was involved in "evil things," having caused many people to suffer. She would now accept the possibility of resolving her karmic debts and spiritually develop, which also gradually improves her current life experiences: initially, she would only work in marginal conditions and feel homesick. At that time, she founded a Spiritist group in the German town of Karlsruhe, which she still supports from a distance. Finally, she received German citizenship and secured employment, and, moving to Munich, she became a member of GEEAK in 2009. She completed a naturopath training with a focus on psychology and, for some time, worked in a psychiatric hospital where she concluded that many patients would not belong there because she would perceive them as mediums instead of mentally ill persons. She decided to support them with joint prayers and conversations on spiritual aspects, but the psychiatric medical staff disliked it and perceived her aspirations as counter-productive and dismissed her. Currently, she works twice a week as a volunteer in a psycho-social care cooperative of the state governmental healthcare provision and Christian institutions. She declares that she mainly tries to "generate happiness," for example, by drumming and dancing, so that participants develop a new sense of life quality and interact with others. As in Spiritist centers, she would bring bottles of water to charge spiritually and share it at the end of her sessions without mentioning its implications for Spiritist practice and knowledge. Her mediumship skills would help her detect energetic-spiritual issues in people, but instead of instructing them in Spiritist terms, she would sit, talk, and pray with them. Regardless of any denomination or ideology, she takes it as her task to create a protective space for people to reflect and resolve their problems, to develop, and to transform as spiritual beings. However, another task would be to guide the medium- ship training of the "German group" within GEEAK to provide essential lessons on theory and practice, as Germans would lack basic knowledge (Interview 16 May 2017).

In conclusion, Sandra practices an approach highly contested at GEEAK, that is, the implementation of Spiritist knowledge and practice into German healthcare systems and an attempt to further develop it as a modality of CAM. She does not discuss it ideologically but adapts it according to her environment, accepting socio-cultural differences as markers of diversifica- tion instead of exclusiveness. It was her example that, at the end of my research, became the starting point for me to consider general insights on the dynamics of Spiritist translocal transformation in the context of health, illness, and healing and, particularly, the diversification of mental healthcare.

Practices of Transformation – Transformation of Practices

Healing Cooperation of Spiritism, biomedicine, and psychiatry is a trans- local phenomenon, but how it is enacted varies in different localities according to their socio-cultural and health-political context. The examples of Dr. Wilhelm, Dr. Hermann, and Dr. Claudionor offer several aspects for comparison of how Spiritist practices complement other healthcare models and how they adapt to their particular environments. It even implies the interconnection of "terrestrial" and "spiritual" localities: concepts of mediumship and obsession are central to all Spiritist practices. They not only serve as explanatory models (cf. Kleinman 1988a,b) or idioms of distress (cf. Nichter 1981), but the mediums-as-therapists "incorporate" external agencies; externalized causes of affliction are resolved with the support of other external forces. This perspective corresponds to the idea that healing mediums are spiritually healed persons themselves and now utilize their experiences to help others. With Paulo and Marcus, it is evident that they suffer from some illness, and all three mediums declare that they do experience relief and some sort of "making sense" in their practices of care.

In Chapter 2, I have already indicated that the Brazilian healthcare system lacks sufficient infrastructure to organize sustained treatment, especially for psychiatric and chronic patients. It is a bifurcate system of state-financed primary care and additional private health plans for those who can afford them. The primary official *Sistema Única de Saúde* (SUS, "Single Health System") promises free treatment to anyone, but it lacks resources. Patients wait for weeks and sometimes even months to be attended, often only receiving marginal treatment and still having to pay for particular diagnostics and medication.[4] Naturally, it is a particularly problematic challenge for economically disadvantaged members of society who are not exclusively but primarily attracted by "spirit doctors" located in their environment and practicing without charging. Other patients even come from more distant localities, but almost all have in common that they have experienced unsuccessful therapy approaches. Therefore, I argue that in contrast to complementary healing cooperation between Spiritism and cosmopolitan (psychiatric) healthcare, as described in Chapters 3 and 4, these practices do not merely complement but substitute non-existent public (mental) healthcare infrastructures. The mediums of Dr. Claudionor (Marcus) and Dr. Hermann (Paulo) are not health professionals themselves but still seek possibilities on how to engage with "terrestrial" medicine: one is supporting the implementation of networks with charitable medical professionals; the other utilizes phytotherapeutic knowledge. Dr. Alexandre/Wilhelm takes a further step: he does not just engage in supporting patients without any therapy success within the public healthcare system; he intends to contribute a spiritual perspective to cosmopolitan medicine. From this angle, they may be simultaneously interpreted as counter-clinics and counter-models to failed health policies. They reveal a certain tendency in the health-seeking behavior of adepts who do not just seek CAM but the integration of "spiritual" aspects into therapy. In this regard, the age average of adepts is interesting: whereas the older generation of Spiritists in Marília tends to engage with "traditional" practices of phytotherapy of Dr. Hermann, the younger ones apply to "modern" discourses on chakras and "energies" provided by Dr. Wilhelm which derive from Buddhist and New Age systems of knowledge, currently influencing health practices all over the world (cf. Heelas 2011). On the other hand, Spiritists in an Afro-Brazilian environment such as in Itabuna show less scruples in integrating entities like *caboclos* or *preto velhos* into their practices, which are usually linked to the practices of *Candomblé* and *Umbanda*. It might be a form of adaption to the cultural context and a strategy to attract Afro-Brazilian adepts, an interpretation that also applies to Dr. Claudionor's declared aim of implementing community meetings with *capoeira* and *samba* performances. However, it also displays local conflicts based on divergent ideological predispositions: in São Paulo, Spiritists tend to deny reciprocal relationships with spirits that are deemed undeveloped and primitive (and especially those related to Afro-Brazilian culture; cf. Kurz 2013, see Chapter 2); in Bahia, Spiritists of any denomination (*Candomblé*, *Umbanda*, Kardecism) are defying attempts of Evangelical/Pentecostal agencies to disturb and denounce their practices as "demonic." It appears that the competition between Spiritists and Evangelicals in Itabuna implies reframing delineations, discourses, and methods for the sake of addressing as many adepts as possible, even though the strategic aims of the opposing agencies could not diverge more: whereas Evangelical institutions are mainly interested in material profit (cf. Riveira 2016), I illustrated that Spiritists are seeking integration and mutual support in non-materialistic terms. Further, even though Greenfield (1987), Hess (1995), and Theissen (2009) claim to observe a continuation of paternalistic structures in Brazilian Spiritism that would serve the quest for power and political influence (see Chapter 2), I did not observe or perceive any stated intentions.[5]

However, conflicts do not reduce to quarrels Spiritists have with external institutions; even within Spiritism, appropriate technologies regarding health-care and spiritual engagement are highly contested. FEB propagates "internal reform" and "study of the doctrine" as ultimate resources of health and well-being and advises against mediumship training of acutely afflicted patients. Furthermore, they deny any practices of medium healers, that is, "spirit doctors." Members of AME and ABRAPE argue differently, pointing at the positive effects of these practices in psychological and "energetic-bodily" terms.

Apart from these ideological divergences, my case studies reveal experiences of a chronic crisis (cf. Vigh 2008) and structural violence (cf. Farmer 2002), and a performative metacommentary and criticism addressing the inequalities and insufficiencies of Brazilian (mental) healthcare. Not only do Spiritists step in where the public health system fails, but they also "copy" certain aspects, such as long waiting hours and marginal resources, with the slight difference that related experiences are transformed: patients receive food, attention, and care which they often miss in official health institutions. Specifically, the effect of *feeling* being attended at all seems to count. Marcus/ Dr. Claudionor revealed to me that even when treatment is solely spiritual, they would act like "regular medical professionals" to have people trust in the treatment: a white coat, band-aids, or a dose of "fluidized water" would already help someone who had never experienced proper attendance and treatment at all.

This observation takes me to the question of how far the Aesthetics of Healing in terms of performativity, hospital mimicry, and other sensory aspects resemble or vary from Spiritist healing practices discussed in Chapters 3 and 4. One year after I participated in his treatment practices, I met Dr. Alexandre again and shared my personal experiences throughout his sessions, including feelings of dizziness, altered states of sensory perception, and headaches. He was very sympathetic and stressed the energetic aspects of therapy and my mediumship capacities, suggesting that once I felt all of that, I would understand more than many of his adepts and clients. He complained that one of the biggest problems would be people's belief in miracles, which implies the expectation of an immediate healing experience. This popular delusion would support performative practices of distraction and suggestion, addressing cultural representations, that is, traditions, symbols, and experiences that patients are accustomed to within the official healthcare system: long waiting hours, reading Spiritist literature (instead of news or gossip magazines), or listening to lectures (instead of watching television on a screen often installed in Brazilian waiting halls) but also the spatial, temporal, and performative structures of treatment with doctors' offices, consultations, therapy staff, pharmacies, surgeries, fragrances, devices, patients' files, etc. He and his colleagues would use this "masquerade" to have people accept it as therapeutic. However, apart from this "trick," they would act as scientific as their "terrestrial" counterparts, exploring spiritual and energetic aspects of affliction and initializing patients' self-healing capacities: "We initiate transformation on cognitive and energetic levels" (Interview 13 Feb. 2017).

In this regard, they even apply to general global processes of medical transfer, hybridization, and diversification, displaying the integration of phytotherapy (for an older generation) and oriental "energetic" approaches (for a younger generation). The majority of patients do not seem aware of these implications and, as I argue in Chapters 3 and 4, it appears to mainly be the aesthetical/sensory aspect of care that is of importance here, not only in the symbolical-performative sense of "being attended," "integrating into a social peer-group," or "triggering imagination," but providing a space of reflection and relaxation. Practices of manipulating the sensory perception of participants by listening to voices that frame their experiences, such as in lectures, prayers, and mediumistic messages, are as immanent as the speaking skills of the lecturers and other speakers: they initiate and intensify internal perceptional processes. Discourse on energies and herbal remedies and the performative "hospital mimicry" might support this experience cognitively, but the treatment mainly consists of a transformation of (self-) perception on a sensory level that does not necessarily lead to therapy success in terms of a cure but at least to a healing experience in terms of developing coping strategies. It includes the affirmation of a Spiritist habitus, which in many patients leads to regular participation in Spiritist practices to help others (see Chapter 3). The modalities of these technologies of the self (cf. Foucault 1988b) might vary in different localities and adapt to their environments, but they resemble in their manipulation of sensory/bodily modes of perception. This is also true for the German example: practices at GEEAK resemble those within the Spiritist centers in Brazil so far that they promote lectures, study groups, mediumship training, energetic treatment, and fraternal care framed by prayers and quotations from the Spiritist literature. As in Brazil, directing participants' attention to voices is predominant, aims at shifting perception, and initiates self-reflection and adjustment. How these practices are implemented varies to a certain degree in different contexts regarding an ongoing appropriation and adaptation of Spiritist practices to their socio-cultural and health-political environments, including conflicts on cultural belonging and interpretations of sovereignty. In both Brazilian and German settings, distress experiences are central to the decision to approach and engage with Spiritist practices.

Related explanatory models may be more prominent in Brazil but are not restricted to national or cultural boundaries. Spiritual agencies, energetic treatment, and personal transformation are aspects of diverse global healing practices that might locally differ in their form but intersect in their content (cf. Littlewood 2000). Spiritist approaches to (mental) healthcare gained importance in 20th-century Brazil but were rooted in European practices of the 19th century (see Chapter 2). Despite being ignored in European scientific discourse for over a century, they have never completely disappeared (cf. Sawicki 2016). In the 21st century, progressing Brazilian transmigration and translocally acting Spiritist networks promote their revitalization in Germany. This dynamic includes contests on political questions of identity and belonging, separations of "religion" and "science" in the German healthcare system, and giving space to cooperation, integration, adaption, and hybridization. The German healthcare system is confronted with an increasing request for spiritual healing practices and their integration not as parallel medical systems but as integral factors of diversification of (mental) healthcare.

Cultural resources of religious and therapeutic practices support the immigrants' integration into a new cultural system (cf. Eichler 2008; Huschke 2013; Thiesbonenkamp-Maag 2014). This is partly true for Kardecism in Germany, and the discussion on the integration of spiritual aspects into a national healthcare system devoid of cultural connotations does not only reflect a debate on political restrictions regarding CAM but also identity politics and their negotiation: approximately one-third of GEEAK consists of German members or Brazilians with a long history as transmigrants in Germany. These postulate a "de-Brazilianization" of Spiritism because they experience practices at GEEAK as too religiously connotated and not in line with their "scientific-philosophical" attitude. Apart from this discourse on the "rationality" of Spiritism and its importance for healthcare and well-being, they are quarreling on language and "socio-cultural" adaption in a way so common in German debates on "integration," initiating the separation of the group in December 2017. Giving way to the new project *Weg der Nächstenliebe* ("Path of Charity"), the members' objective is to utilize their (Brazilian) Spiritism networks and to adapt Spiritist knowledge and practice to the German context. Some plan to seek rapport with therapists to explore possibilities of health-related initiatives and, e.g., AME member Moreira (cf. 2013; see Chapter 1) increasingly implements lectures and courses in Germany, promoting the (re)distribution of Spiritist knowledge, practice, and approaches to (mental) healthcare.

Notes

1   I would not call it a cure because, until today, I perceive a certain "weakness" in the area of my back that had suffered from a disc prolapse years before when I still worked as a nurse. However, ever since, I have hardly felt any pain.
2   For the discussion on consciousness in Brazilian mediumship, see Schmidt (2015).
3   For example, on my first day of participation, the rampage of München (22 July 2016) that took place only a few days earlier was discussed from a Spiritist perspective.
4   This is, by the way, an increasing tendency in the German healthcare system, too.
5   Quite the opposite, Spiritists all over Brazil tend to summon a final battle between "good" and "evil" agencies (cf. Xavier 1939) that may be envisioned in contemporary health policies in Brazil.

Chapter 6

Conclusion
Voices of Good Sense

A critique has been levelled at modern medicine which goes something like this: Medical practice, though it has gained much over the last century in clinical efficacy, has lost something as well. Most importantly, it has progressively lost the human touch. Patients are often treated in a depersonalized, even dehumanized, fashion within the modern health-care system. Their suffering is not heard and responded to; their wishes are not incorporated fully into treatment decisions; their resources for self-healing are not called into play.

(Leder 1992: 1)

Leder stresses the fact that this critique encompasses perspectives of patients, healers, and other participants of therapy processes alike: patients feel being treated like a "piece of meat" or just "another interesting case: poked, prodded, examined, tested, diagnosed, medicated, but not treated as a person with respect and consideration" (ibid.), and while medical ethicists address a lack of effectively informed consent and patient autonomy, healthcare practitioners lament overpressures that force them into such impersonal care. Critical theoreticians and self-declared "holistic" practitioners locate asymmetric power relations in invasive technologies that characterize medical practice corrupted by capitalism, bureaucracy, and institutionalized interest groups (ibid.: 1ff). Overall, these perspectives dismiss a paradigm of modern medicine that produces distorted concepts of Self and the human body as a machine to be fixed instead of a living entity with unique relations to and interactions with its environment (ibid.: 25).

By imperial networks, this model has been transported worldwide, but parallelly, cultural resistance and postcolonial negotiations have produced spaces of medical diversity and medical revivalism that shape and complement contemporary Public Health policies in their attempt to cushion structural violence and manage social and spiritual relations as essential for health and well-being. Particularly regarding mental health, they counteract suffering, stigmatization, forced isolation, medicalization, marginalization, corrupted infrastructures, and unequal access to therapeutic

DOI: 10.4324/9781032637167-6

resources. Bhabha (1994) proposes the concept of Third Space to frame cultural contests as interstices where individual and interpersonal coping strategies are negotiated and developed. Stressing the performativity of related dynamics, he interprets contact zones as liminal spaces of interaction where practices are transformed and (re)created. They are charged with meanings and (re)interpreted, and a cultural "Other" may infiltrate without necessarily confronting local customs (ibid.: 3). Applying this perspective to therapeutic practices, Baer et al. (2013) state that contemporary realities of medical diversity reveal dynamics of cultural hybridization but are still hegemonically controlled by biomedical and psychiatric discourse.

Contemporary developments in Brazil reveal a contradictory reality, where cosmopolitan medicine, psychiatry, and Spiritism seem to shape each other on eye level mutually. Sharing common European roots may facilitate this apparent symmetric relationship (see Chapter 2). However, they have divergently developed, and only at the edge of the 21st century, they have started to embrace again – particularly in Brazil but subsequently worldwide, too. One interpretation for the increasing interest in spiritual healing practices may address patients' agency as a crucial aspect of therapy. Recurrent arguments imply that biomedicine alienates patients from doctors, their ailments, and their understanding of treatment processes, whereas alternative healing practices empower them and take their individual experiences seriously. However, such a perspective again connotes approaches in biomedicine, psychiatry, and/or CAM as homogenous and separated practices – an idea that anthropological concepts of diversity and hybridization refute. My investigation of (Brazilian) Spiritism and its entanglements with mental healthcare has aimed to explore diversifications, pluralities, and transformations in heterogeneous contexts. It adds to psychiatric and anthropological research on relationships between religious/spiritual knowledge and practice, societal values, divergent explanatory models of mental health and illness, and psychiatric nosology and treatment. In a comparable approach, Koss-Chioino (2003) observes "[...] an ongoing discussion in psychiatry regarding the meaning and dynamics of phenomena labeled 'dissociative states' and 'altered states of consciousness' such as visions, trance, and possession by spirits [...]" (ibid.: 126). Referring to Carl Gustav Jung and in accordance with Spiritist concepts, she discusses to what extent neuroses and psychoses may be potentially constructive ways to deal with the intrusion of abnormal "unconscious material into the ego" (ibid.), an experience that among Spiritists would constitute engagements with spirits (ibid.: 132).

Apart from my sensory-aesthetic focus on related practices, my analysis has revealed Healing Cooperation and Translocal Relations as central aspects of the diversification and hybridization of psychiatric medical discourse, contributing to new territories in medical anthropology that deny systemic and culture-specific approaches but instead develop perspectives investigating global circulations of both biomedical and so-called alternative healing practices in translocal spaces. They arise from global migratory dynamics, patients' or therapists' consideration of public health and welfare systems as inadequate, and their consequent search for alternatives in a diversified global health market. It is particularly true for mental healthcare as a subject to increasing pathologization, medicalization, and, therefore, economization of alleged socially deviant behavior, its experience, communication, and negotiation. Such controversies manifest in agendas emphasizing the protection of human rights and community-based care, as well as the establishment of counter-clinics, where spaces of well-being constitute alternative treatment methods. My example of the German Spiritist center GEEAK illustrates that such spiritually supported initiatives and counter-drafts are not to be understood as culture-bound phenomena but approaches that will increasingly contribute to the (trans)local diversification and negotiation of mental healthcare.

My argument is that these processes of mental healthcare diversification involve aspects of sensory work and emplacement, creating hybrid, socially and culturally localized therapeutic spaces of (self-)care, empathy, and experiences of healing as a transformation of self. They transcend dichotomous constructions of body and mind that have largely characterized psychiatric practices; still, dimensions of experience and embodied sensation of mental affliction and care remain white spots on many maps of therapeutic landscapes, and related bodily/sensory responses remain black boxes. My contribution intends to fill this epistemological gap and suggests the concept of Aesthetics of Healing as an approach that may deepen and expand our understanding of crucial dynamics for the diversification of mental health/care at the intersection of Global Health, CAM, local policies, and translocal spiritual engagement. For the case of Spiritism, I have illustrated that the essence of the therapeutic cooperation of Spiritists and psychiatrists is the production of an alleged healthy Spiritist habitus via sensory techniques and manipulations triggering interoceptive processes comparable to contemplative practices of, e.g., mindfulness (cf. Farb et al. 2015).

The medium of voice (cf. Dolar 2006; Basu 2017a,b, 2018) appears to be particularly important here: Spiritist practices emphasize the voices of spirits, mediums, presenters, lecturers, and devotees while other sensory stimuli are reduced. This practice aimed at contemplation causes shifts in physical-sensory and cognitive processes of perception. Spiritist spaces contrast general predominant visual-aesthetic and physical-expressive sensory codes with the sole impression of auditory experiences and thus create a tangible alternative reality to the everyday experience of a busy, noisy environment (see Chapter 4). However, "healing" is also fused with moral values of individualization, e.g., patients should learn to take responsibility for their spiritual development and ultimately also for others so that aspects of self-care and care merge (cf. Thiesbonenkamp-Maag 2014; see Chapter 3).

This approach appears to be of increasing relevance due to reissued attempts of Global Health agencies to delimit biomedicine from religious and Indigenous institutions. The contemporary experience of the COVID-19 pandemic has well illustrated that biomedical lobbies neglect alternative approaches, conditioning and disciplining humanity for their alleged benefit (cf. LeMonde 2021) while at the same time increasing Global Health inconsistencies and injustices (cf. Manderson et al. 2021). As discussed elsewhere,[1] I do not intend to analyze the so-called Corona measures since 2020, but I argue for considering experiential aspects of medical interventions. To stick to the example, social distancing and isolation throughout the lockdowns caused many to suffer mentally,[2] adding to an age of depression (cf. Furedi 2004; Ehrenberg 2010).[3] In this regard, some patients, therapists, and medical anthropologists demand more aesthetic engagement and agency in care and treatment (cf. Kurz 2019) and integration of related approaches with healthcare systems that remain to be framed by policies of inequality and impossibilities (cf. Thompson 2020; Hatzikidi & Dullo 2021; Kurz 2022).[4]

A challenging result of my investigation is the role of Spiritist institutions as actors antithetical to Public Health policies and economic dynamics. During my research, HEM changed from a psychiatry to a polyclinic due to a realignment of Brazilian health policy (see Chapters 2 and 3). As part of the deinstitutionalization reform, mere psychiatric hospitals have ceased being funded by the public health system *Sistema Única de Saúde* (SUS), which is why, with donations and volunteer work, a surgical station was built in 2015/2016 to maintain public co-financing with the status of a polyclinic. In Itabuna, on the other hand, the *Centro Espírita Claudionor de Carvalho* (CECC), as already noted, replaces the inadequate infrastructures of public healthcare devoid of any financial interests. All processes are financed through donations in currency or kind or the sale of Spiritist books. The same is true for the German Spiritist center (see Chapter 5), which, as a charitable institution, contrasts other upcoming profit-oriented spiritual healing institutions.

The Brazilian psychiatry deinstitutionalization reform of the early 21st century, the insufficient efforts of various Brazilian governments to improve the public healthcare system, and the recent political and economic crises have resulted in marginal medical supply, especially for the disadvantaged members of Brazilian society and particularly in the mental health sector. Spiritists and other religious-spiritual institutions fill the gap in cooperation with dedicated health professionals. Healing Cooperation of Spiritism, biomedicine, and psychiatry thus seems to be a local phenomenon unique to Brazil's social-cultural-political contexts. How does it correspond to the situation in Germany?

In general, many Brazilian immigrants appear to perceive Spiritist centers in Germany as "places of well-being" (cf. Ferraro & Barletti 2016) where they can reflect on daily experiences and find social support within a "Brazilian environment" as a community of people with similar experiences. Practices of Spiritist centers in Brazil and Germany resemble each other except, of course, the use of the German language. Participants are aware of the psycho-social health aspect that addresses an inner transformation and dedication to new spiritual practices in ways of self-healing. They experience relief from a disturbing condition that could have easily resulted in severe mental health problems due to specific forms of structural violence. Many experience integration by participating in a protective "Brazilian retreat" and sometimes a more challenging mixed peer group. Furthermore, German and more "progressive" Brazilian members are dedicated to continuously disseminating Spiritist doctrine for healing practices within the German culture. The case studies (see Chapter 5) provide several crucial insights for analyzing Spiritism as an example of the translocal, transnational, and transcultural transfer of healing cooperation from one context to another. First, in both cultural frames, experiences of distress play a specific role in the decision to engage in Spiritism and a life-long dedication to it. Second, Spiritist explanatory models may be very prominent in Brazil but are not limited to its national borders. Concepts of spirit obsession, energy treatment, and personal transformation through spiritual devotion are global phenomena that may differ in their local form but resemble in content (cf. Littlewood 2000).

From the perspective of medical anthropology, discussing the diversification of mental healthcare with the matrix of the transnational expansion of Spiritist healing practices does not mean arguing for their universal validity but assuming that they are – just like practices in cosmopolitan medicine – universally transformable, integrable, and contestable according to patients' needs, experiences, expectations, and resources. Spiritists address contested realms of healing at the intersection of scientific and spiritual knowledge, postulating "holistic" approaches toward health, care, and well-being. As my case studies illustrate, Spiritist mental healthcare is not a homogenous field; apart from the adaptation to specific socio-cultural contexts and conflicts with outside forces, different orientations contest within the particular networks of Spiritism. AME aims at the scientific investigation of Spiritist techniques, explores extraneous approaches such as energetic healing, and integrates patients in mediumship practices. On the other hand, FEB acts more like a religious institution that aims at the moral development of its adepts.

Here, I must also provide some space for critical voices. Parallel to my field research, my colleague Sabrina Del Sarto investigated the Spiritist engagement of *moradores* at HEM, that is, those long-term patients who live there as an act of charity of the Spiritist administration. They complain that they are forced to participate in the daily morning lectures and the *passe* (Del Sarto & Langdon 2019), thus contradicting my observation of the voluntary engagement of patients. One explanation for these divergent observations may be that the long-term patients I worked with were mainly in the private health insurance ward, which may reflect the inequalities in Brazilian healthcare, even within Spiritist institutions. Whereas I have focused on the healing cooperation between psychiatric, biomedical, and Spiritist institutions, the asymmetries among different groups of patients and between them and their therapists must be further explored in future research projects.

Another critical aspect in the moralization of adepts is the interpretation of human affliction and suffering as a necessary evil that, in my opinion, results in the relativization, if not justification, of racism, gender discrimination, sexual exploitation, and structural violence. Of all my research situations, it has become most apparent to me in Silvia's ESDE course on the introduction to Spiritism (see Chapter 3): Silvia always provides a space for discussion but concludes by imposing her interpretation of the Spiritist doctrine. Since she always asks my opinion, we sometimes contest on certain questions and develop extensive discussions, for example, when she replicates Xavier's (1938: 47ff) message that the enslavement of Africans and their integration into Brazilian society have been necessary for the spiritual growth of both, slaves and masters: people would have to learn lessons not about revenge or compensation but about (re)interpreting suffering and affliction as a path toward spiritual well-being and progress. It is an example of how, in Spiritism, explanatory models of cause and effect, even though presented and performed as what we may call a "science mimicry," do not only juxtapose a cosmopolitan academic perspective but caricature and contradict it: it is undeniable that historical dynamics sustainably *did* influence religious/spiritual practices, frames, and discourse in Brazil, but to deduct that, therefore, it was *necessary*, appears apologetic and opportunistic to me. On another occasion, Silvia mentions the example of rape and declares that in many cases, the female victims might have been promiscuous and reckless males in previous lives and now would have to experience "the other side of the coin." The rationality behind it is that there are no clear-cut categories of "victims" and "culprits" within a cosmology that communicates spiritual progress throughout many reincarnations. Still, justifying criminal and immoral behavior as a "necessity" instead of a "side effect" of human progress is a giant pill to swallow, even though I respect the idea of promoting forgiveness and future orientation instead of revenge and regress. The danger is a systematic tolerance of aggression in line with denying the right of resistance.

Apart from the engagement with healing, these aspects add an unsavory flavor to Kardecism as a political institution supporting the oppression of certain parts of society (cf. Theissen 2009; see Chapter 2). Another problematic topic is homosexuality, which Silvia, in line with the Spiritist doctrine, describes as an instance of men understanding their femininity (and vice versa). Therefore, with proper spiritual development, gay people could recover from their unnatural behavior as a resolvable identity issue. I am aware of my bias and the ethical claim of participant observers not to influence "their field" more than necessary. However, even many Brazilians would consider these ideas discriminatory, apologetic, and unethical. Especially as I consider her a good friend who has helped me where she could throughout my research, Silvia's response to my doubts left me even more negatively affected: "We can only understand what we can understand, and even if it looks like a terrible injustice and crime against humanity, it might serve a higher spiritual purpose, and we should not question our spiritual guides but trust in their knowledge and insight" (Session 16 Dec. 2015).

I perceive a considerable gap between this apologetic and moralistic cognitive approach of Kardecist discourse and aesthetic Spiritist care practices. It applies to (self-)responsibility, but I wonder how that might help a client/patient who has become a victim of structural violence, racism, or sexual discrimination. I have, therefore, interviewed several participants of Silvia's course to learn more about their motives, expectations, and insights they would link to their participation. One of them is Danilo, a 23-year-old student raised Catholic but frequenting Spiritist centers since the age of seventeen. It was not a health crisis that brought him there but his homosexuality, and he has been looking for answers that "the church" cannot provide. He declares that it has been vital to him to understand his homosexuality as a process of self-knowledge and as a means to become attached to the Spiritist doctrine and accept and understand it as a personal challenge to be resolved. He tells me that even though he has suffered from intolerance and stigmatization, he can now better handle his homosexuality and social reactions to it. However, in the homophobic environment of the Brazilian countryside, I doubt that he will receive sustained alleviation as long as he believes that *he* has to learn something (Interview 23 Jan. 2016).

I unraveled these contradictions and paradoxes throughout my discussions with Silvia, but she always has concluded that I must learn more before I can understand it. Back then, I considered it an arrogant, disrespectful, and lop-sided argument that would question my rational and critical capacities. It took me some time to understand that Silvia did not want to attack me or prove me wrong but to develop a different approach that is not so much based on widespread models of human cognition and psychology but aims at the level of affection without explicitly addressing it. She does not preach or teach; she provides a frame where individuals can reinterpret their experiences and do so in a way that they acknowledge their agency and feel empowered. Tereza's case may serve as another last example: she grew up in an Evangelic community but left "her church" at the age of thirty-three and stresses that it was a relief as she would not have to listen anymore to sermons on "hell, sin, and punishment" and to witness evangelic pastors controlling, disciplining, and exploiting their adepts in moral, bodily, and economic terms. Instead of supporting followers to develop and focus on care and charity spiritually, Evangelicals would promote and reproduce a model of (self-)salvation that orientates toward a materialist economic model of exploitation, bondage, patronage, and clientage (cf. Strickon & Greenfield

1972). With the diagnosis of depression, she had been a patient of HEM several times and now states that medical treatment with antidepressants and spiritual practices would complement each other: one would tranquilize her, and the other would provide hope. With Spiritism, Tereza would learn that God does not punish her for misbehavior but would provide opportunities for self-knowledge and the insight that "hell is here, and we create it." The study group provides relief from work and her daily worries, and she perceives it as enriching to understand and reflect on her experiences within a peer group. In the future, she wants to learn more about mediumship, especially to understand her daughter's and her sixteen-year-old grandson's related experiences: "All of this is the proof that this is real, that we come back, that there is life after death. It is important to know that we will meet again." Tereza also stresses the importance of energetic healing:

> I love it; it makes me feel great because I come here tired from work, but after the study, I receive the *passe* and return home calmly. I sleep well, and my husband mentions how well I am doing, enjoying that I am not going off on him for anything. I get rid of my worries. When I feel bad, I drink fluidified water during the week; it is pure energy.
>
> (Interview 25 Jan. 2016)

I suggest further exploring these implications of (spiritual/religious) mental healthcare on an interdisciplinary basis that considers the concept of Aesthetics of Healing as a tool to investigate therapeutic settings' experiential and sensory aspects. As Thompson (2020) puts it, we must explore the different ways in which people think and practice care and accordingly adjust our methodological and theoretical considerations of approaching, investigating, and interpreting them. Studying the aesthetics of mental healthcare in Brazilian Spiritism means developing a notion of the "art of care" (ibid.: 38), envisioning attentiveness to those who are unattended (ibid.: 41), and, even more critically, valuing the work of those that take care of Selves and Others.

Notes

1   Curare 43(2020)1–4 & 44(2021)1–4 on the Corona Diaries I & II, see https://agem.de/en/curare/archive/.
2   See https://boasblogs.org/curarecoronadiaries/.
3   As a study program coordinator and lecturer for over a decade, I have never received so many requests from students to postpone their examinations due to a diagnosis of depression. This development has continued even after reimplementing physical participation in seminars and lectures.
4   To provide one prominent example, the public healthcare systems in many countries, including Brazil and Germany, differentiate between public and private health insurance, granting disparate access to health resources.

References

Adams, Vincanne, Mona Schrempf & Sienna R. Craig (eds. 2011): *Medicine between Science and Religion. Explorations on Tibetan Grounds*. New York: Berghahn.

Alberti, Sonia (2003): *Crepúsculo da Alma. A Psicologia no Brasil no Século XIX*. Rio de Janeiro: Contra Capa.

Alex, Gabriele (2018): The Relevance of Embodiment for Health-Seeking Behavior. In: Philipp Zehmisch et al. (eds.): *Soziale Ästhetik, Atmosphäre, Medialität. Beiträge aus der Ethnologie*. Münster: LIT. pp. 143–149.

Amarante, Paulo (2018): Prefácio. In: Mônica Nunes & Tiago Pires Marques (eds.): *Legitimidades da Loucura. Sofrimento, Luta, Criatividade e Pertença*. Salvador: EDUFBA. pp. 7–9.

Araújo, Annette (1991): Herr Doktor, es sind die Nerven. Zur Relevanz "Traditioneller" Erklärungsmodelle in der Schulmedizin am Beispiel Brasiliens. In: Robert Wiedersheim et al. (eds.): *Traditionelle Heilsysteme und Religionen. Ihre Bedeutung für die Gesundheitsversorgung in Asien, Afrika und Lateinamerika*. Saarbrücken: Dadder. pp. 157–167.

Associação Medico-Espírita (eds. 2009): *Saúde e Espiritismo*. 4th Edition. São Paulo: AME.

Aubrée, Marion & François Laplantine (2009[1990]): *A Mesa, o Livro e os Espíritos. Gênese, Evolução e Atualidade do Movimento Social Espírita entre França e Brasil*. Maceió: EdUFAL.

Aureliano, Waleska d.A. & Vânia Z. Cardoso (2015): Spiritism in Brazil. From Religious to Therapeutic Practice. In: Cathy Gutierrez (ed.): *Handbook of Spiritualism and Channeling*. Leiden: Brill. pp. 275–293.

Baer, Hans A., Merrill Singer & Ida Susser (2013): *Medical Anthropology and the World System. Critical Perspectives*. 3rd Edition. Santa Barbara: Praeger.

Bahia, Joana (2014): Under the Berlin Sky. Candomblé on German Shores. *Vibrant* 11(2): 326–369.

Barnes, Linda L. (2011): New Geographies of Religion and Healing. States of the Field. *Practical Matters* 4: 1–82.

Barrow, Logie (1986): *Independant Spirits. Spiritualism and English Plebeians 1850–1910*. London: Routledge & Kegan Paul.

Basu, Helene (2009): Contested Practices of Control. Psychiatric and Religious Mental Health Care in India. *Curare* 32(1+2): 28–39.

Basu, Helene (2014a): Davā and Duā. Negotiating Psychiatry and Ritual Healing of Madness. In: Harish Naraindas et al. (eds.): *Asymmetrical Conversations. Contestations, Circumventions, and the Blurring of Therapeutic Boundaries*. Oxford: Berghahn. pp. 162–199.

Basu, Helene (2014b): Listening to Disembodied Voices. Anthropological and Psychiatric Challenges. *Anthropology & Medicine* 21(3): 325–342.
Basu, Helene (2017a): The Voice of Crisis (Comment). In: Martina Wagner-Egelhaaf (ed.): *Stimmen aus dem Jenseits. Ein interdisziplinäres Projekt/Voices from Beyond. An Interdisciplinary Project.* Würzburg: Ergon. pp. 98–100.
Basu, Helene (2017b): Voices of Possession. In: Martina Wagner-Egelhaaf (ed.): *Stimmen aus dem Jenseits. Ein interdisziplinäres Projekt/Voices from Beyond. An Interdisciplinary Project.* Würzburg: Ergon. pp. 253–266.
Basu, Helene (2018): The Mediality of the Voice in Local Islamic Practices. In: Philipp Zehmisch et al. (eds.): *Soziale Ästhetik, Atmosphäre, Medialität. Beiträge aus der Ethnologie.* Münster: LIT. pp. 127–131.
Basu, Helene, Roland Littlewood & Arne S. Steinforth (eds. 2017): *Spirit & Mind. Mental Health at the Intersection of Religion & Psychiatry.* Berlin: LIT.
Beaudevin, Claire & Laurent Pordié (2016): Diversion and Globalization in Biomedical Technologies. *Medical Anthropology* 35(1): 1–4.
Bell, Catherine (1992): *Ritual Theory, Ritual Practice.* New York: Oxford University Press.
Bell, Catherine (2006): Embodiment. In: Jens Kreinath et al. (eds.): *Theorizing Rituals. Issues, Topics, Approaches, Concepts.* Leiden: Brill. pp. 533–543.
Bell, Sarah L. et al. (2018): From Therapeutic Landscape to Healthy Spaces, Places, and Practices. A Scoping Review. *Social Science & Medicine* 196: 123–130.
Bernardo, Marcia B. & Andréia d.C. Garbin (2011): A Atenção à Saúde Mental Relacionada ao Trabalho no SUS. Deasafios e Possibilidades. *Revista Brasileira de Saúde Ocupacional* 36(123): 103–117.
Bezerra de Menezes, Adolfo (1920[1897]): *A Loucura sob Novo Prisma.* São Paulo: FEB.
Bhabha, Homi K. (1994): *The Location of Culture.* New York: Routledge.
Bhugra, Dinesh (ed. 1996): *Religion and Psychiatry. Context, Consensus and Controversies.* London: Routledge.
Biehl, João (2005): *Vita. Life in a Zone of Social Abandonment.* Photographs by Torben Eskerod. Berkeley: University of California Press.
Biehl, João (2018): Care and Disregard. In: Mônica Nunes & Tiago P. Marques (eds.): *Legitimidades da Loucura. Sofrimento, Luta, Criatividade e Pertença.* Salvador: EDUFBA. pp. 249–283.
Black, Steven P. (2018): The Ethics and Aesthetics of Care. *Annual Review of Anthropology* 47: 79–95.
Bourdieu, Pierre (1977[1972]): *Outline of a Theory of Practice.* Cambridge: University Press.
Botega, Neury. J. (2002): Psychiatric Units in Brazilian General Hospitals. A Growing Philanthropic Field. *International Journal of Social Psychiatry* 48: 97–102.
Bowie, Fiona (2016): Negotiating Blurred Boundaries. Ethnographical and Methodological Considerations. In: George Chryssides & Stephen Gregg (eds.): *The Insider/Outsider Debate. New Perspective in the Study of Religion.* Sheffield: Equinox. pp. 110–129.
Brabec de Mori, Bernd (2002): *Ikaro. Medizinische Gesänge der Ayawaska-Zeremonie im Peruanischen Regenwald. Diplomarbeit Musikwissenschaft.* Wien: Universität Wien.
Brabec de Mori, Bernd (2015): *Die Lieder der Richtigen Menschen. Musikalische Kulturanthropologie der Indigenen Bevölkerung im Ucayali-Tal, Westamazonien.* Dissertation Ethnomusikologie. Wien: Universität Wien.
Bragdon, Emma (2004): *Kardec's Spiritism. A Home for Healing and Spiritual Evolution.* Woodstock: Lightening Up.

Bragdon, Emma (2012a): Introduction. In: Emma Bragdon (ed.): *Spiritism and Mental Health. Practices from Spiritist Centers and Spiritist Psychiatric Hospitals in Brazil*. London: Singing Dragon. pp. 10–20.

Bragdon, Emma (2012b): Case Studies of Those with Serious Diagnoses. In: Emma Bragdon (ed.): *Spiritism and Mental Health. Practices from Spiritist Centers and Spiritist Psychiatric Hospitals in Brazil*. London: Singing Dragon. pp.55–69.

Bragdon, Emma (2012c): The Spiritist Psychiatric Hospital of Porto Alegre. In: Emma Bragdon (ed.): *Spiritism and Mental Health. Practices from Spiritist Centers and Spiritist Psychiatric Hospitals in Brazil*. London: Singing Dragon. pp. 82–87.

Brandt, Klaus (2014): *Wissenschaft und Religion in Mesmerismusdiskursen des 19. Jahrhunderts. Ein Beitrag zum Religionsbegriff und zur Entstehung moderner Spiritualität*. Münster: Monsenstein & Vannerdat.

Bretfeld, Sven (2012): Dynamiken der Religionsgeschichte. Lokale und Translokale Verflechtungen. In: Michael Stausberg (ed.): *Religionswissenschaft*. pp. 423–433.

Brickell, Katherine & Ayona Datta (eds. 2011): *Translocal Geographies. Spaces, Places, Connections*. Farnham: Ashgate.

Brody, Eugene B. (1973): *The Lost Ones. Social Forces and Mental Illness in Rio de Janeiro*. New York: International University Press.

Brown, Diana (1986): *Umbanda. Religion and Politics in Urban Brazil*. Michigan: UMI.

Brown, Diana (1999): Power, Invention, and the Politics of Race. Umbanda Past and Future. In: Larry Crook & Randal Johnson (eds.): *Black Brazil. Culture, Identity and Social Mobilization*. Los Angeles: University of California Press.

Budden, Ashwin (2010): *Moral Worlds and Therapeutic Quests. A Study of Medical Pluralism and Treatment-Seeking in the Lower Amazon*. Dissertation. San Diego: University of California, Department of Anthropology and Cognitive Science.

Bull, Michael & Jon P. Mitchell (2015): Introduction. In: Michael Bull & Jon P. Mitchell (eds.): *Ritual, Performance, and the Senses*. London: Bloomsbury. pp. 1–10.

Burns Coleman, Elisabeth & Kevin White (eds. 2010): *Medicine, Religion, and the Body*. Leiden: Brill.

Caldwell, Kia L. (2017): *Healthy Equity in Brazil. Intersections of Gender, Race and Policy*. Urbana: University of Illinois Press.

Camargo, Cândido P.F. (1961): *Kardecismo e Umbanda*. São Paulo: Pioneira.

Cantalice, Tiago (2011): O Melhor do Brasil é o Brasileiro! Corpo, Identidade, Desejo e Poder. *Sexualidad, Salud y Sociedad* 7: 69–102.

Cartwright, Elizabeth & Jerome W. Crowder (2017): Dissecting Images. Multimodal Medical Anthropology. *Medical Anthropology* 36(6): 515–518.

Cerqueira, Vera C. & Margarida L. Felgueiras (2018): Pedagogias da Alteridade. Perspectivas sobre a Emoção de Lidar: Manuela Malpique e Nise da Silveira. *Revista da Educação Pública* 27(66): 927–949.

Chau, Adam Y. (2008): The Sensorial Production of the Social. *Ethnos* 73(4): 485–504.

Ciello, Fernando J. (2013): *Saúde Mental, Loucura e Saberes. Reforma Psiquiatrica, Interações e Identidades em uma Clínica-Dia*. Curitiba: UFPR: Master Thesis.

Ciello, Fernando J. (2019): *A Vida do Diagnóstico. Práticas Terapêuticas e Movimentos em uma Clínica-Dia. Dissertation in Social Anthropology*. Florianópolis: UFSC.

Claro, Izaias (2008): *Depressão. Causas, Conseqüências e Tratamento*. Matão: Clarim.

Classen, Constance (1993): *Worlds of Sense. Exploring the Senses in History and Across Cultures*. London: Routledge.

Classen, Constance (1999): Other Ways of Wisdom. Learning Through the Senses Across Cultures. *International Review of Education* 45(3+4): 269–280.

Cohen, Mark (2017): A Systematic Approach to Understanding Mental Health and Services. *Social Science & Medicine* 191: 1–8.

Comaroff, Jean & John Comaroff (2012): *Theory from the South, or How Euro-America is Evolving Toward Africa*. Boulder: Paradigm.

Conselho Federal de Psicologia et al. (2018): *Relatório da Inspeção Nacional em Comunidades Terapêuticas – 2017*. Brasília: Conselho Federalde Psicologia; Mecanismo Nacional de Prevenção e Combate à Tortura; ProcuradoriaFederal dos Direitos do Cidadão / Ministério Público Federal.

Crabtree, Adam (2015): Mesmerism and the Psychological Dimension of Mediumship. In: Cathy Gutierrez (ed.): *Handbook of Spiritualism and Channeling*. Leiden: Brill. pp. 9–31.

Critchley, Hugo D. & Sarah N. Garfinkel (2017): Interoception and Emotion. *Current Opinion in Psychology* 17: 7–14.

Csordas, Thomas J. (1990): Embodiment as a Paradigm for Anthropology. *Ethos* 18(1): 5–47.

Csordas, Thomas J. (1993): Somatic Modes of Attention. Cultural *Anthropology* 8(2): 135–156.

Csordas, Thomas J. (1994): *The Sacred Self. A Cultural Phenomenology of Charismatic Healing*. Berkeley: University of California Press.

Csordas, Thomas J. (2002): *Body, Meaning, Healing*. New York: Palgrave Macmillan.

Csordas, Thomas J. (ed. 2009): *Transnational Transcendence. Essays on Religion and Globalization*. Berkeley: University of California Press.

Csordas, Thomas J. (2017): Psychiatry and the Sweat Lodge. Therapeutic Resources for Native American Adolescents. In: Helene Basu et al. (eds.): *Spirit & Mind. Mental Health at the Intersection of Religion & Psychiatry*. Berlin: LIT. pp. 127–140.

da Glória Cohn, Maria (2010): Interessengruppen, soziale Bewegungen und Akteure der Zivilgesellschaft. In: Sérgio Costa et al. (eds.): *Brasilien Heute. Geographischer Raum, Politik, Wirtschaft, Kultur*. 2nd Edition. Frankfurt/Main: Vervuert. pp. 235–244.

DaMatta, Roberto (1997): *A Casa e a Rua. Espaço, Cidadania, Mulher e Morte no Brasil*. 5th Edition. Rio de Janeiro: Rocco.

Davis, Elizabeth A. (2018): Global Side Effects. Counter-Clinics in Mental Health Care. *Medical Anthropology* 37(1): 1–16.

Dein, Simon & Roland Littlewood (2007): The Voice of God. *Anthropology & Medicine* 14(2): 213–228.

Del Sarto, Sabrina M. & E. Jean Langdon (2019): Healing Efficacy and Subjectivity among Long-Term Residents in a Spiritist Asylum. *Curare* 42(3+4): 93–106.

de Oliveira, Sérgio F. (2009): Cristais da Glândula Pinealö. Semicondutores Cerebrais? In: Associação Medico Espírita (eds.): *Saúde e Espiritismo*. 4th Edition. São Paulo: AME. pp. 93–100.

de Olivieira, Célio Alan Kardec de, Jairo Avelar, Wanderlev Soares de Oliveira & Wander Luiz de Lemos (2001): *Depressão e Mediunidade. Sob o Ponto de Vista do Doutrina Espírita, da Psiquiatria e da Psicologia*. Belo Horizonte: AME.

Desjarlais, Robert R. (1992): *Body and Emotion. The Aesthetics of Illness and Healing in the Nepal Himalayas*. Philadelphia: University of Pennsylvania Press.

Desjarlais, Robert R. & C. Jason Throop (2011): Phenomenological Approaches in Anthropology. *Annual Review of Anthropology* 40: 87–102.

Devereux, George (1980): *Basic Problems of Ethnopsychiatry*. Chicago: University Press.

Dilthey, Petra (1993): *Krankheit und Heilung im brasilianischen Spiritismus. Der Geistchirurg Dr. med. Edson Queiroz im Kontext spiritistisch-medizinischer Medizinkultur.* München: Akademischer Verlag.

Dolar, Mladen (2006): *A Voice and Nothing More.* Cambridge: MIT.

Douglas, Mary (1970): *Natural Symbols. Explorations in Cosmology.* London: Barrie & Rockliff.

Downey, Greg (2015): The Importance of Repetition. Ritual as a Support to Mind. In: Michael Bull & Jon P. Mitchell (eds.): *Ritual, Performance, and the Senses.* London: Bloomsbury. pp. 45–61.

Downey, Greg (2016): Sensory Enculturation and Neuroanthropology. The Case of Human Echolocation. In: Joan Y. Chiao et al. (eds.): *The Oxford Handbook of Cultural Neuroscience.* Oxford: University Press. pp. 41–55.

Dox, Donnalee (2016): *Reckoning with Spirit in the Paradigm of Performance.* Ann Arbor: University of Michigan Press.

Duncan, Janet (2012): What Spiritist Centers offer outside Brazil. In: Emma Bragdon (ed.): *Spiritism and Mental Health. Practices from Spiritist Centers and Spiritist Psychiatric Hospitals in Brazil.* London: Singing Dragon. pp. 249–256.

Egnew, Thomas R. (2005): The Meaning of Healing. Transcending Suffering. *Annals of Family Medicine* 3(3): 255–262.

Ehrenberg, Alain (2010[1998]): *The Weariness of the Self. Diagnosing the History of Depression in the Contemporary Age.* Montreal & Kingston: McGill-Queen's University Press.

Eichler, Katja J. (2008): *Migration, Transnationale Lebenswelten und Gesundheit. Eine qualitative Studie über das Gesundheitshandeln von Migrantinnen.* Wiesbaden: VS.

Eisenstadt, Shmuel N. (ed. 2017[2002]): *Multiple Modernities.* New York: Routledge.

Eller, Jack D. (2019): *Psychological Anthropology for the 21st Century.* London: Routledge.

Engler, Steven & Ênio Brito (2016): Afro-Brazilian and Indigenous-Influenced Religions. In: Bettina E. Schmidt & Steven Engler (eds.): *Handbook of Contemporary Religions in Brazil.* Leiden: Brill. pp. 142–169.

Espirito Santo, Diana (2015): *Developing the Dead. Mediumship and Selfhood in Cuban Espiritismo.* Gainesville: University of Florida Press.

Farb, Norman, Jennifer Daubenmier, Cynthia J. Price, Tim Gard, Catherine Kerr, Barnaby D. Dunn, Anne Carolyn Klein, Martin P. Paulus & Wolf E. Mehling (2015): Interoception, Contemplative Practice, and Health. *Frontiers in Psychology* 6(763): 1–26.

Farmer, Paul (2002): On Suffering and Structural Violence. A View from Below. In: Joant Vincent (ed.): *The Anthropology of Politics. A Reader in Ethnography, Theory, and Critique.* Malden: Blackwell. pp. 424–437.

Farmer, Paul (2005): *Pathologies of Power. Health, Human Rights, and the New War on the Poor.* Berkeley: University of California Press.

Ferraro, Emilia & Juan P.S. Barletti (2016): Placing Wellbeing. Anthropological Perspectives on Wellbeing and Place. *Anthropology in Action* 23(3): 1–5.

Figge, Horst H. (1973): *Geisterkult, Besessenheit und Magie in der Umbanda-Religion Brasiliens.* Freiburg: Alber.

Foucault, Michel (1988a[1961]): *Madness and Civilization. A History of Insanity in the Age of Reason.* New York: Vintage Books.

Foucault, Michel (1988b): Technologies of Self. In: Luther H. Martin et al. (eds.): *Technologies of the Self. A Seminar with Michel Foucault.* London: Tavistock. pp. 16–49.

Foucault, Michel (1995[1975]): *Discipline and Punish. The Birth of the Prison.* New York: Vintage Books.

Franco, Divaldo P. (2009[2003]): *Aspectos Psiquiátricos e Espirituais nos Transtornos Emocionais.* Salvador: LEAL.

Franco, Divaldo P. (2010): *A Obsessão e o Movimento Espírita.* Santo André: EBM.

Furedi, Frank (2004): *Therapy Culture. Cultivating Vulnerability in an Uncertain Age.* London: Routledge.

Gaonkar, Dilip P. (ed. 2001): *Alternative Modernities.* Durham: Duke University Press.

Gattaz, Wagner F. & Hannes Stubbe (1981): Trends in der Psychiatrischen Versorgung in Brasilien. *Social Psychiatry* 16: 199–204.

Geertz, Clifford (1973[1966]): *The Interpretation of Cultures.* New York: Basic Books.

Geertz, Clifford (1974): From the Native's Point of View. On the Nature of Anthropological Understanding. *Bulletin of the American Academy of Arts and Sciences* 28(1): 26–45.

Gibbs, Raymond W. Jr. (2005): *Embodiment and Cognitive Science.* Cambridge: University Press.

Giddens, Anthony (1979): *Central Problems in Social Theory. Action, Structure and Contradiction in Social Analysis.* London: MacMillan.

Giovanella, Ligia & Marcelo F.d.S. Porto (2004): *Gesundheitswesen und Gesundheitspolitik in Brasilien.* Arbeitspapier Nr. 25. Frankfurt/Main: Institut für Medizinische Soziologie.

Giumbelli, Emerson (1994): *O Cuidado dos Mortos. Uma Historia da Condenação e Legitimação do Espiritismo.* Rio de Janeiro: Arquivo Nacional.

Giumbelli, Emerson (2003): O "Baixo Espiritismo" e a Historia dos Cultus Mediúnicos. *Horizontes Antropológicos* 9(19): 247–281.

Giumbelli, Emerson (2008): A Presença do Religioso no Espaço Público. Modalidades no Brasil. *Religião & Sociedade* 28(2): 80–101.

Goode, Erich (2019): *Deviant Behavior.* 12th Edition. New York: Routledge.

Gottowik, Volker (2010): Transnational, Translocal, Transcultural. Some Remarks on the Relations between Hindu-Balinese and Ethnic Chinese in Bali. *Sojourn* 25(2): 178–212.

Goulart, Maria S.B. & Flávio Durães (2010): A Reforma e os Hospitais Psiquiátricos. Histórias da Desinstitucionalização. *Psicologia e Sociedade* 22(1): 112–120.

Greene, Jeremy, Marguerite T. Basilico, Heidi Kim & Paul Farmer (2011): Colonial Medicine and its Legacies. In: Paul Farmer et al. (eds.): *Reimagining Global Health. An Introduction.* Berkeley: University of California Press. pp. 33–73.

Greenfield, Sidney M. (1987): The Return of Dr. Fritz. Spiritist Healing and Patronage Networks in Urban, Industrial Brazil. *Social Science & Medicine* 24(12): 1095–1108.

Greenfield, Sidney M. (1992): Spirits and Spiritist Therapy in Southern Brazil. A Case Study of an Innovative Syncretic Healing Group. *Culture, Medicine & Psychiatry* 16: 23–51.

Greenfield, Sidney M. (2004): Treating the Sick with Morality Play. The Kardecist-Spiritist Disobsession in Brazil. In: Don Handelman & Galina Lindquist (eds.): *Ritual in its Own Right. Exploring the Dynamics of Transformation.* New York: Berghahn. pp. 174–194.

Greenfield, Sidney M. (2008): *Spirits with Scalpels. The Culturalbiology of Religious Healing in Brazil.* Walnut Creek: Left Coast.

Greenfield, Sidney M. (2016): The Alternative Economics of Alternative Healing. Faith-Based Therapies in Brazil's Religious Marketplace. *Research in Economic Anthropology* 36: 315–336.

Gruner-Domić, Sandra (2005): *Latinas in Deutschland. Eine Ethnologische Studie zu Migration, Fremdheit und Identität.* Münster: Waxmann.

Guedes, Simoni L. (1974): Umbanda e Loucura. In: Gilberto Velho (ed.): *Desvio e Divergência. Uma Crítica da Patologia Social.* Rio de Janeiro: Zahar. pp. 82–98.

Gutierrez, Cathy (2015): Introduction. In: Cathy Gutierrez (ed.): *Handbook of Spiritualism and Channeling.* Leiden: Brill. pp. 1–6.

Hacking, Ian (1995): The Looping Effects on Human Kinds. In: Dan Sperber et al. (eds.): *Causal Cognition. A Multi-Disciplinary Debate.* Oxford: University Press. pp. 351–383.

Hageman, Joan H., Julio F.P. Peres, Alexander Moreira-Almeida, Leonarda Caixeta, Ian Wickramasekera II & Stanley Krippner (2010): The Neurobiology of Trance and Mediumship in Brazil. In: Stanley Krippner & Harris L. Friedmann (eds.): *Mysterious Minds. The Neurobiology of Psychics, Mediums and Other Extraordinary People.* Santa Barbara: Praeger. pp. 85–111.

Halliburton, Murphy (2009): *Mudpacks and Prozac. Experiencing Ayurvedic, Biomedical and Religious Healing.* Walnut Creek: Left Coast.

Hatzikidi, Katerina & Eduardo Dullo (eds. 2021): *A Horizon of (Im)Possibilities. A Chronicle of Brazil's Conservative Turn.* London: CLACS.

Heelas, Paul (2011): *Spirituality in the Modern World. Within Religious Tradition and Beyond.* London: Routledge.

Hess, David J. (1987): Religion, Heterodox Science and Brazilian Culture. *Social Studies of Science* 17(3): 465–477.

Hess, David J. (1991): *Spirits and Scientists. Ideology, Spiritism, and Brazilian Culture.* University Park: PSU.

Hess, David J. (1995): Hierarchy, Heterodoxy, and the Construction of Brazilian Religious Therapies. In: David J. Hess & Roberto A. DaMatta (eds.): *The Brazilian Puzzle. Culture on the Borderlands of Western Culture.* New York: Columbia University Press: pp. 180–206.

Hinton, Devon, David Howes & Laurence J. Kirmayer (2008): Towards a Medical Anthropology of Sensations. Definitions and Research Agendas. *Transcultural Psychiatry* 45(2): 142–162.

Hollan, Douglas & C. Jason Throop (2008): Whatever happened to Empathy? Introduction. *Ethos* 36(4): 385–401.

Hörbst, Viola & Angelika Wolf (2014): ARV and ARTs. Medicoscapes and the Unequal Place-Making for Biomedical Treatments in Sub-Saharan Africa. *Medical Anthropology Quarterly* 28(2): 182–202.

Howes, David (2003): *Sensual Relations. Engaging the Senses in Culture and Social Theory.* Ann Arbor: University of Michigan Press.

Howes, David (ed. 2005): *Empire of the Senses. The Sensual Culture Reader.* Oxford: Berg.

Howes, David (ed. 2009): *The Sixth Sense Reader.* Oxford: Berg.

Howes, David (2015): Sensation and Transmission. In: Michael Bull & Jon P. Mitchell (eds.): *Ritual, Performance, and the Senses.* London: Bloomsbury. pp. 153–166.

Hsu, Elizabeth (2008a): Medical Pluralism. In: Harald K. Heggenhougen & Stella Quah (eds.): *International Encyclopedia of Public Health.* Vol IV. Amsterdam: Elsevier. pp. 316–321.

Hsu, Elisabeth (2008b): The Senses and the Social: An Introduction. *Ethnos* 73(4): 433–443.

Hüwelmeier, Gertrud & Kristine Krause (eds. 2010): *Traveling Spirits. Migrants, Markets, and Mobilities.* New York: Routledge.

Huizer, Gerrit (1987): Indigenous Healers and Western Dominance. Challenge for Social Scientists? *Social Compass* 34: 415–436.

Hume, Lynne (2007): *Portals. Opening Doorways to Other Realities through the Senses.* Oxford: Berg.

Huschke, Susann (2013): *Kranksein in der Illegalität. Undokumentierte LateinamerikanerInnen in Berlin. Eine Medizinethnologische Studie.* Bielefeld: Transcript.

IBGE (2000): *Censo Demográfico 2000. Caraterísticas Gerais da População: Resultados da Amostra.* Rio de Janeiro: IBGE.

IBGE (2011): *Censo Demográfico 2010. Características da População e dos Domicílios: Resultados do Universo.* Rio de Janeiro: IBGE.

Incayawar, Mario, Ronald Wintrob & Lise Bouchard (eds. 2009): *Psychiatrists and Traditional Healers. Unwitting Partners in Global Mental Health.* Chichester: Wiley-Blackwell.

Ingold, Tim (2000): *The Perception of the Environment. Essays in Livelihood, Dwelling and Skill.* London: Routledge.

Ingold, Tim (2001): Beyond Art and Technology. The Anthropology of Skill. In: Michael B. Schiffer (ed.): *Anthropological Perspectives on Technology.* Albuquerque: University of New Mexico Press. pp. 17–31.

Ingold, Tim (2013): Religious Perception and the Education of Attention. Religion. *Brain & Behavior* 4(2): 156–158.

Inhorn, Maria C. & Emily A. Wentzell (eds. 2012): *Medical Anthropology at the Intersections. Histories, Activisms, and Futures.* Durham: Duke University Press.

Isaia, Arthur C. (2010): Transe Mediúnico e Norma Médica na Faculdade de Medicina do Rio de Janeiro da Primeira Metade do Século XX. O Olhar de Xavier de Oliveira. *Esboços* 17(23): 31–50.

Jabert, Alexander (2011): Popular Strategies for Identification and Treatment of Insanity in the First Half of the Twentieth Century. An Analysis of Medical Charts from the Uberaba Spiritist Asylum. *História, Ciências, Saúde* 18(1): 1–15.

Jain, Sumeet & David M.R. Orr (2016): Ethnographic Perspectives on Global Mental Health. *Transcultural Psychiatry* 53(6): 685–695.

Jenkins, Janis H. (2015): *Extraordinary Conditions. Culture and Experience in Mental Illness.* Oakland: University of California Press.

Johannessen, Helle & Imre Lázár (eds. 2006): *Multiple Medical Realities. Patients and Healers in Biomedical, Alternative and Traditional Medicine.* New York: Berghahn.

Kabat-Zinn, Jon (2003): Mindfulness-Based Interventions in Context. Past, Present, and Future. *Clinical Psychology: Science and Practice* 10(2): 144–156.

Kapchan, Deborah (2009): Learning to Listen. The Sound of Sufism in France. *The World of Music* 51(2): 65–89.

Kapferer, Bruce (1983): *A Celebration of Demons. Exorcism and the Aesthetics of Healing in Sri Lanka.* Bloomington: Indiana University Press.

Kardec, Allan (1986 [1861]): *The Mediums' Book.* Rio de Janeiro: FEB.

Kardec, Allan (1996 [1857]): *The Spirits' Book.* Rio de Janeiro: FEB.

Kardec, Allan (2008 [1864]): *The Gospel according to Spiritism.* Brasilia: ISC.

Keane, Webb (2000): Voice. *Journal of Linguistic Anthropology* 9(1+2): 271–273.

Kirmayer, Laurence J. (1989a): Cultural Variations in the Response to Psychiatric Disorders and Emotional Distress. *Social Science & Medicine* 29(3): 327–339.

Kirmayer, Laurence J. (1989b): Psychotherapy and the Cultural Concept of the Person. *Santé, Culture, Health* 6(3): 241–270.

Kirmayer, Laurence J. (2006): Beyond the "New Cross-Cultural Psychiatry." Cultural Biology, Discursive Psychology and the Ironies of Globalization. *Transcultural Psychiatry* 43(1): 126–144.

Kirmayer, Laurence J. (2008): Empathy and Alterity in Cultural Psychiatry. *Ethos* 36(4): 457–474.

Kirmayer, Laurence J. (2014): Medicines of the Imagination. Cultural Phenomenology, Medical Pluralism, and the Persistence of Mind-Body Dualism. In: Harish Naraindas et al. (eds.): *Asymmetrical Conversations. Contestations, Circumventions, and the Blurring of Therapeutic Boundaries.* New York: Berghahn. pp. 26–55.

Kirmayer, Laurence J. (2015): Mindfulness in Cultural Context. *Transcultural Psychiatry* 52(4): 447–469.

Kleinman, Arthur (1988a): *Rethinking Psychiatry. From Cultural Category to Personal Experience.* New York: Free Press.

Kleinman, Arthur (1988b): *The Illness Narratives. Suffering, Healing, and the Human Condition.* New York: Basic Books.

Kleinman, Arthur (2012): Medical Anthropology and Mental Health. Five Questions for the Next Fifty Years. In: Maria C. Inhorn & Emily A. Wentzell (eds.): *Medical Anthropology at the Intersections.* Durham: Duke University Press. pp. 116–128.

Klinkhammer, Gritt & Eva Tolksdorf (eds., 2015): *Somatisierung des Religiösen. Empirische Studien zum Rezenten Religiösen Heilungs- und Therapiemarkt.* Bremen: Universität.

Knoblauch, Hubert (2009): *Populäre Religion. Auf dem Weg in eine Spirituelle Gesellschaft.* Frankfurt/Main: Campus.

Kohrt, Brandon & Emily Mendenhall (eds. 2015): *Global Mental Health. Anthropological Perspectives.* Walnut Creek: Left Coast.

Kolesch, Doris & Sybille Krämer (ed. 2006): *Stimme.* Frankfurt/Main: Suhrkamp.

Koss-Chioino, Joan D. (2003): Jung, Spirits and Madness. Lessons for Cultural Psychiatry. *Transcultural Psychiatry* 40: 164–180.

Kraatz, Elisabeth S. (2001): The Structure of Health and Illness in a Brazilian Favela. *Journal of Transcultural Nursing* 12: 173–178.

Krause, Kristine, Gabriele Alex & David Parkin (2012): Medical Knowledge, Therapeutic Practice, and Processes of Diversification. MMG Working Paper 12(11): Göttingen: Max-Planck Institute for the Study of Religious and Ethnic Diversity.

Kriesel, Stephan (2001): *Der Körper als Paradigma. Leibesdiskurse in Kultur, Volksreligiosität und Theologie Brasiliens.* Luzern: Exodus.

Krippner, Stanley & Emma Bragdon (2012): Contributions of Brazilian Spiritist Treatments to the Global Improvement of Mental Health Care. In: Emma Bragdon (ed.): *Spiritism and Mental Health: Practices from Spiritist Centers and Spiritist Psychiatric Hospitals in Brazil.* London: Singing Dragon.

Kurz, Helmar (2013): *Performanz und Modernität im brasilianischen Candomblé. Eine Interpretation.* Hamburg: Kovač.

Kurz, Helmar (2015): "Depression is not a Disease. It is a Spiritual Problem." Performance and Hybridization of Religion and Science within Brazilian Spiritist Healing Practices. *Curare* 38(3): 173–191.

Kurz, Helmar (2017): Diversification of Mental Health. Brazilian Kardecist Psychiatry and the Aesthetics of Healing. *Curare* 40(3): 195–206.

Kurz, Helmar (2018a): Transcultural and Transnational Transfer of Therapeutic Practice. Healing Cooperation of Spiritism, Biomedicine, and Psychiatry in Brazil and Germany. *Curare* 41(1+2): 39–53.

Kurz, Helmar (2018b): Affliction and Consolation. Mediumship and Spirit Obsession as Explanatory Models within Brazilian Kardecist Mental Health-Care. In: Mônica Nunes & Tiago P. Marques (eds.): *Legitimidades da Loucura. Sofrimento, Luta, Criatividade e Pertença.* Salvador: EDUFBA. pp. 129–154.

Kurz, Helmar (ed. 2019): The Aesthetics of Healing. Working with the Senses in Therapeutic Spaces. *Curare* 42(3+4).

Kurz, Helmar (2022): Politics and Aesthetics of Care. Chronic Affliction and Spiritual Healing in Brazilian Kardecism. In: Andrew R. Hatala & Kerstin Roger (eds.): *Spiritual, Religious, and Faith-Based Practices in Chronicity. An Exploration of Mental Wellness in Global Context*. London: Routledge. pp. 76–99.

Kurz, Helmar (2023): Sensory Ethnography and Anthropology of Mediumship. Exploring Brazilian Spiritist Practices in (Mental) Well-Being and Health/Care. In: Emily Pierini et al. (eds.): *Other Worlds, Other Bodies. Embodied Epistemologies and Ethnographies of Healing*. New York: Berghahn. pp. 211–229.

Kutschera, Franz von (1988): *Ästhetik*. Berlin: Gruyter.

Laderman, Carol & Marina Roseman (eds. 1996): *The Performance of Healing*. New York: Routledge.

Landmann-Szwarcwald, Celia & James Macinko (2016): A Panorama of Health Inequalities in Brazil. *International Journal for Equity in Health* 15: 174–176.

Laplantine, Francois (2015): *The Life of the Senses. Introduction to a Modal Anthropology*. London: Bloomsbury.

Latour, Bruno (1996): On Actor-Network-Theory. A Few Clarifications Plus More than a Few Complications. *Soziale Welt* 47: 369–381.

Leder, Drew (1992): Introduction. In: Drew Leder (ed.): *The Body in Medical Thought and Practice*. Dordrecht: Kluwer. pp. 1–12.

Leibing, Annette (1995): *Blick auf eine Verrückte Welt. Kultur und Psychiatrie in Brasilien*. Münster: LIT.

Leibing, Annette (2007): Much More than Medical Anthropology. The Healthy Body and Brazilian Identity. In: Francine Saillant & Serge Genest (eds.): *Medical Anthropology. Regional Perspectives and Shared Concerns*. Malden: Blackwell. pp. 58–70.

LeMonde, Julia (2021): Exploring Regimes of "Truth" during COVID-19. *Curare* 44(1–4): 95–106.

Leonardi, Jeff & Bettina E. Schmidt (2020): Introduction. In: Bettina E. Schmidt & Jeff Leonardi (eds.): *Spirituality and Wellbeing. Interdisciplinary Approaches to the Study of Religious Experience and Health*. Sheffield: Equinox. pp. 1–15.

Levi-Strauss, Claude (1963): *Structural Anthropology*. New York: Basic Books.

Lewgoy, Bernardo (2001): Chico Xavier e a Cultura Brasileira. *Revista de Anthropologia* 44(1): 53–116.

Lewgoy, Bernardo (2006a): Incluídos e Letrados: Reflexões sobre a Vitalidade do Espiritismo Kardecista no Brasil Atual. In: Faustino Teixeira & Renata Menezes (eds.): *As Religiões no Brasil. Continuidades e Rupturas*. Petrópolis: Vozes. pp. 173–188.

Lewgoy, Bernardo (2006b): Representações de Ciência e Religião no Espiritismo Kardecista: Antigas e Novas Configurações. *Civitas* 6(2): 151–167.

Lewgoy, Bernardo (2008): A Transnacionalição do Espiritismo Kardecista Brasileiro. Uma Discussão Initial. *Religião e Sociedade* 28(1): 84–104.

Lewis, Maureen (2006): Governance and Corruption in Public Health Care Systems. *Center for Global Development*. Working Paper 78: 1–57.

Littlewood, Roland (2000): Psychiatry's Culture. In: Vieda Skultans & John Cox (eds.): *Anthropological Approaches to Psychological Medicine. Crossing Bridges*. London: Kingsley. pp. 66–93.

Long, Debbi, Cynthia Hunter & Sjaak van der Geest (2008): When the Field is a Ward or a Clinic. Hospital Ethnography. *Anthropology & Medicine* 15(2): 71–78.

Lott, Micah (2016): Agency, Patiency, and the Good Life. The Passivities Objection to Eudaimonism. *Ethical Theory & Moral Practice* 19(3): 773–786.

Lüddeckens, Dorothea & Monika Schrimpf (eds. 2018): *Medicine, Religion, Spirituality. Global Perspectives on Traditional, Complementary, and Alternative Healing*. Bielefeld: Transcript.

Luhrmann, Tanya M. (2010): What Counts as Data? In: James Davies & Dimitrina Spencer (eds.): *Emotions in the Field. The Psychology and Anthropology of Fieldwork Experience*. Stanford: University Press. pp. 212–238.

Luz, Madel T. (1979): *As Instituições Médicas no Brasil. Instituição e Estratégia de Hegemonia*. Rio de Janeiro: Graal.

Luz, Madel T. (2014): *As Instituições Médicas no Brasil*. 2nd Edition. Porto Alegre: UNIDA.

Lynch, Darrell (2005): Patient Preparation and Perceived Outcomes of Spiritist Healing in Brazil. *Anthropology of Consciousness* 15(1): 10–41.

Machleidt, Wielant (2013): *Migration, Kultur, und Psychische Gesundheit. Dem Fremden Begegnen*. Stuttgart: Kohlhammer.

Maggie, Yvonne (1992): *Medo de Feitiço. Relações entre Magia e Poder no Brasil*. Rio de Janeiro: Arquivo Nacional.

Maggie, Yvonne (2007): Medo de Feitiço 15 Anos Depois. "A Ilusão da Catequese" Revisitada. In: Olivia M.G.d. Cunha & Flávio d.S. Gomes (eds.): *Quase-Cidadão. Histórias e Antropologias da Pos-Emanicipação no Brasil*. Rio de Janeiro: FGV. pp. 347–376.

Manderson, Lenore, Nancy J. Burke & Ayo Wahlberg (eds. 2021): *Viral Loads. Anthropologies of Urgency in the Time of Covid-19*. London: UCL.

Mateus, Mario D., Jair J. Mari, Pedro G.G. Delgado, Naomar Almeida-Filho, Thomas Barrett, Jeronimo Gerolin, Samuel Goihman, Denise Razzouk, Jorge Rodriguez, Renata Weber, Sergio B. Andreoli & Shekhar Saxena (2008): The Mental Health System in Brazil. Policies and Future Challenges. *International Journal of Mental Health Systems* 2(12): 1–8.

Maués, Raymundo H. (2003): Bailando com o Senhor. Técnicas Corporais de Culto e Louvor (O Êxtase e o Transe como Técnicas Corporais). *Revista de Antropologia* 46(1): 9–40.

Mauss, Marcel (1975): *Soziologie und Anthropologie*. Band 2. München: Hanser.

Mauss, Marcel (1985[1938]): A Category of Human Mind. The Notion of Person, the Notion of Self (translated by W.D. Halls). In: Michael Carrithers et al. (eds.): *The Category of the Person. Anthropology, Philosophy, History*. Cambridge: University Press. pp. 1–25.

McCarthy-Jones, Simon (2012): *Hearing Voices. The Histories, Causes and Meanings of Auditory Verbal Hallucinations*. Cambridge: University Press.

Messias, DeAnne K.H. (2002): Transnational Health Resources, Practices, and Perspectives. Brazilian Immigrant Women's Narratives. *Journal of Immigrant Health* 4(4): 183–200.

Ministério da Saúde (2004): *Saúde Mental no SUS. Os Centros de Atenção Psicosocial*. Brasília: Ministério da Saúde.

Ministério da Saúde (2007): *Saúde Mental no SUS. Acesso ao Tratamento e Mudança do Modelo de Atenção. Relatório de Gestão 2003–2006*. Brasília: Ministério da Saúde.

Ministry of Health (2008): *National Policy on Integrative and Complementary Practices of the SUS*. Brasília: Ministry of Health.

Monroe, John W. (2015): *Crossing Over. Allan Kardec and the Transnationalisation of Modern Spiritualism*. In: Cathy Gutierrez (ed.): Handbook of Spiritualism and Channeling. Leiden: Brill. pp. 248–274.

Montero, Paula (1985): *Da Doença à Desordem. A Magia na Umbanda*. Rio de Janeiro: Graal.

Moreira, Andrei (2013): *Cura e Autocura. Uma Visão Médico-Espírita*. Belo Horizonte: AME.

Moreira-Almeida, Alexandre & Francisco Lotufo Neto (2005): Spiritist Views of Mental Disorders in Brazil. *Transcultural Psychiatry* 42(4): 570–595.

Motta, Roberto (2005): Body Trance and Word Trance in Brazilian Religion. *Current Sociology* 53(2): 293–308.

Münster, Daniel (2001): *Religionsästhetik und Anthropologie der Sinne*. München: Akademischer Verlag.

Munari, Luciano (2008): *Ectoplasma. Descobertas de um Médico Psiquiatra*. Limeira: Conhecimento.

Nichter, Mark (1981): Idioms of Distress. Alternatives in the Expression of Psychosocial Distress: A Case Study from South India. *Culture, Medicine & Psychiatry* 5: 379–408.

Nichter, Mark (2008): Coming to our Senses. Appreciating the Sensorial in Medical Anthropology. *Transcultural Psychiatry* 45(2): 163–197.

Nichter, Mark (2010): Idioms of Distress Revisited. *Culture, Medicine & Psychiatry* 34: 401–416.

Nissen, Nina & Lenore Manderson (2013): Researching Alternative and Complementary Therapies. Mapping the Field. *Medical Anthropology* 32(1): 1–7.

Noland, Carrie (2009): *Agency and Embodiment. Performing Gestures/Producing Cultures*. Cambridge: Harvard University Press.

Nunes, Mônica & Tiago Pires Marques (2018): Introdução. In: Mônica Nunes & Marques Tiago Pires (eds.): *Legitimidades da Loucura. Sofrimento, Luta, Criatividade e Pertença*. Salvador: EDUFBA. pp. 11–28.

Obst, Helmut (2009): *Reinkarnation. Weltgeschichte einer Idee*. München: Beck.

Paixão Santos, Marcos R. & Mônica de Oliveira Nunes (2011): Território e Saúde Mental. Um Estudo sobre a Experiência de Usuários de um Centro de Atenção Psicosocial, Salvador, Bahia, Brasil. *Interface* 15(38): 715–726.

Parkin, David (2013): Medical Crises and Therapeutic Talk. *Anthropology & Medicine* 20(2): 124–141.

Peluso, Érica d.T.P. & Sérgio L. Blay (2009): Public Beliefs about the Treatment of Schizophrenia and Depression in Brazil. *International Journal of Social Psychiatry* 55: 16–27.

Pierini, Emily (2020): *Jaguars of the Dawn. Spirit Mediumship in the Brazilian Vale do Amanhecer*. New York: Berghahn.

Pierini, Emily & Alberto Groisman (2016): Introduction. Fieldwork in Religion – Bodily Experience and Ethnographic Knowledge. *Journal for the Study of Religious Experience* 2: 1–6.

Pink, Sarah (2009): *Doing Sensory Ethnography*. London: SAGE.

Pink, Sarah (2011): Multimodality, Multisensoriality & Ethnographic Knowing. Social Semiotics and the Phenomenology of Perception. *Qualitative Research* 11(1): 261–276.

Pinto, Luiz A. (2015): Editorial. O Drama da Saúde Mental. *Visão Hospitalar* 4(11): 3.

Pols, Jeannette (2016): Analyzing Social Spaces. Relational Citizenship for Patients leaving Mental Health Care Institutions. *Medical Anthropology* 35(2): 177–192.

Porcello, Thomas, Louise Meintjes, Ana M. Ochoa & David W. Samuels (2010): The Reorganization of the Sensory World. *Annual Review of Anthropology* 39: 51–66.

Porter, Roy (1987): *A Social History of Madness. Stories of the Insane*. London: Phoenix.

Prandi, Reginaldo (2013): *Os Mortos e os Vivos. Uma Introdução ao Espiritismo.* São Paulo: Três Estrelas.

Rabelo, Miriam C.M. (1993): Religião e Cura. Algumas Reflexões sobre a Experiência Religiosa das Classes Populares Urbanas. *Cadernos da Saúde Pública* 9(3): 316–325.

Rabelo, Miriam C.M. (2005): Religião e a Transformação da Experiência. Notas sobre o Estudo das Práticas Terapêuticas nos Espaços Religiosos. *Ilha* 7(1+2): 126–145.

Rabelo, Miriam C.M. & Iara Souza (2003): Temporality and Experience. On the Meaning of *Nervoso* in the Trajectory of Urban Working-Class Women in Northeast Brazil. *Ethnography* 4(3): 333–361.

Rabelo, Miriam C.M., Sueli R. Mota & Claudio R. Almeida (2009): Cultivating the Senses and Giving In to the Sacred. Notes on Body and Experience among Pentecostal Women in Salvador, Brazil. *Journal of Contemporary Religion* 24(1): 1–18.

Redko, Cristina (2003): Religious Construction of a First Episode of Psychosis in Urban Brazil. *Transcultural Psychiatry* 40: 507–530.

Ribeiro, Leonidio & Murillo de Campos (1931): *O Espiritismo no Brasil. Contribuição ao seu Estudo Clinico e Medico-Legal.* São Paulo: Nacional.

Riveira, Paulo B. (2016): Pentecostalism in Brazil. In: Bettina E. Schmidt & Steven Engler (eds.): *Handbook of Contemporary Religions in Brazil.* Leiden: Brill. pp. 117–131.

Rocha, Cristina (2017): *John of God. The Globalization of Brazilian Faith Healing.* Oxford: University Press.

Rodaway, Paul (1994): *Sensuous Geographies. Body, Senses, and Place.* London: Routledge.

Rödiger, Kerstin (2003): *Körper. Vergessene Kategorie der Ethik?.* Münster: LIT.

Ross, Anamaria I. (2012): *The Anthropology of Alternative Medicine.* Oxford: Berg.

Santos, José L. (2004): *Espiritismo. Uma Religião Brasileira.* Campinas: Atomo.

Saraiva, Clara (2010): Afro-Brazilian Religions in Portugal. Bruxos, Priests, and Pai de Santos. *Ethnográfica* 14(2): 265–288.

Sawicki, Diethard (2016): *Leben mit den Toten. Geisterglauben und die Entstehung des Spiritismus in Deutschland 1770-1900.* Paderborn: Schöningh.

Sawodny, Heike (2003): *Die Kardecistische Bewegung in Deutschland. Spiritistische Praxis, Weltbild und Lebenseinstellung.* Hamburg: Universität Hamburg: Master Thesis.

Sayers, Janet (2004): Healing Aesthetics. Kristeva through Stokes. *Theory & Psychology* 14(6): 777–795.

Scharf da Silva, Inga (2004): *Umbanda. Eine Religion zwischen Candomblé und Kardecismus: Über Synkretismus im städtischen Alltag Brasiliens.* Münster: LIT.

Scheper-Hughes, Nancy (1994): Embodied Knowledge. Thinking with the Body in Critical Medical Anthropology. In: Robert Borofsky (ed.): *Assessing Cultural Anthropology.* New York: McGraw-Hill: pp. 229–242.

Scheper-Hughes, Nancy & Margaret M. Lock (1987): The Mindful Body. A Prolegomenon to Future Work in Medical Anthropology. *Medical Anthropology Quarterly* 1(1): 7–41.

Schiller, Nina G., Linda Basch & Cristina S. Blanc (1995): From Immigrant to Transmigrant. Theorizing Transnational Migration. *Anthropology Quarterly* 68(1): 48–63.

Schmidt, Bettina E. (2015): Spirit Mediumship in Brazil. The Controversy about Semi-Conscious Mediums. *Diskus* 17(2): 38–53.

Schmidt, Bettina E. (2016a): *Spirits and Trance in Brazil. An Anthropology of Religious Experience.* London: Bloomsbury.

Schmidt, Bettina E. (2016b): Spirit Possession. In: Bettina E. Schmidt & Steven Engler (eds.): *Handbook of Contemporary Religion in Brazil*. Leiden: Brill. pp. 431–447.

Schmidt, Bettina E. (2017): Varieties of Non-ordinary Experiences in Brazil. A Critical Review of the Contribution of Studies of "Religious Experience" to the Study of Religion. *International Journal of Latin American Religions*. DOI 10.1007/s41603-017-0006-5.

School, Rosa (2015): O Colapso na Saúde Mental. Reforma implantada em 2001 provoca diminuição no número de leitos psiquiátricos no Brasil. *Visão Hospitalar* 4(11):10–13.

Schubert, Cornelius & Ehler Voss (2018): Beyond Dyadic Interactions. An Introduction to the Thematic Issue on Healing Cooperations. *Curare* 41(1+2): 11–16.

Seligman, Rebecca (2005): Distress, Dissociation, and Embodied Experience. Reconsidering the Pathways to Mediumship and Mental Health. *Ethos* 33(1): 71–99.

Seligman, Rebecca (2010): The Unmaking and Making of Self. Embodied Suffering and Mind-Body-Healing in Brazilian Candomblé. *Ethos* 38(3): 297–320.

Seligman, Rebecca (2014): *Possessing Spirits and Healing Selves. Embodiment and Transformation in an Afro-Brazilian Religion*. New York: Palgrave MacMillan.

Seligman, Rebecca, Suparna Choudhury & Laurence J. Kirmayer (2016): Locating Culture in the Brain and in the World. From Social Categories to the Ecology of Mind. In: Joan Y. Chiao et al. (eds.): *The Oxford Handbook of Cultural Neuroscience*. Oxford: University Press. pp. 3–20.

Sharman, Russell (1997): The Anthropology of Aesthetics. A Cross-Cultural Approach. *JASO* 28(2): 177–192.

Sharp, Lynn L. (2006): *Secular Spirituality. Reincarnation in Nineteenth-Century France*. Lanham: Lexington.

Sharp, Lynn L. (2015): Reincarnation. The Path to Progress. In: Cathy Gutierrez (ed.): *Handbook of Spiritualism and Channeling*. Leiden: Brill. pp. 221–247.

Shorter, Edward (1997): *A History of Psychiatry. From the Era of Asylum to the Age of Prozac*. New York: Wiley.

Silva de Almeida, Angélica A., Ana Maria G.R. Oda & Paulo Dalgalarrondo (2007): O Olhar dos Psiquiatras Brasileiros Sobre os Fenômenos de Transe e Possesão. *Revista de Psiquiatria Clínica* 34(1): 34–41.

Skultans, Vieda (2007): *Empathy and Healing. Essays in Medical and Narrative Anthropology*. New York: Berghahn.

Slaby, Jan, Rainer Mühlhoff & Philipp Wüschner (2017): Affective Arrangements. *Emotion Review*: 1–10. DOI: 10.1177/1754073917722214.

Spinu, Marina & Henry Thorau (1994): *Captação. Trancetherapie in Brasilien: Eine Ethnopsychologische Studie über Heilung durch Telepathische Übertragung*. Berlin: Reimer.

Spittler, Gerd (2001): Teilnehmende Beobachtung als Dichte Teilnahme. *Zeitschrift für Ethnologie* 126: 1–25.

Stelzig-Willutzki, Sabina (2012): *Soziale Beziehungen im Migrationsverlauf. Brasilianische Frauen in Deutschland*. Wiesbaden: Springer VS.

Sterzi, Valeria (2011): *Dancing Spirits. Umbanda Healing Practices and the Market of Identity in Cosmopolitan London*. London: University College London: Department of Anthropology. Dissertation.

Stoll, Sandra J. (2002): Religião, Ciência ou Auto-Ajuda? Trajetos do Espiritismo no Brasil. *Revista de Antropologia* 45(2): 361–402.

Stoll, Sandra J. (2003): *Espiritismo à Brasileira*. São Paulo: EDUSP.

Stoll, Sandra J. (2004): Narrativas Biográficas. A Construção da Identidade Espírita no Brasil e sua Fragmentação. *Estudos Avançados* 18(52): 181–199.

Stoll, Sandra J. (2005): O Espiritismo na Encruzilhada. Mediunidade com Fins Lucrativos? *Revista USP* 67: 176–185.

Strathern, Andrew J. & Pamela J. Stewart (1999): *Curing and Healing. Medical Anthropology in Global Perspective*. Durham: Carolina Academic Press.

Strickon, Arnold & Sidney M. Greenfield (eds. 1972): *Structure and Process in Latin America. Patronage, Clientage, and Power Systems*. Albuquerque: University of New Mexico Press.

Stubbe, Hannes (1987): *Geschichte der Psychologie in Brasilien. Von den Indianischen und Afrobrasilianischen Kulturen bis in die Gegenwart*. Berlin: Reimer.

Teixera, Faustion & Renata Menezes (2006): Introdução. In: Faustion Teixera & Menezes Renata (eds.): *As Religiões no Brasil. Continuidades e Rupturas*. Petrópolis: Vozes. pp. 7–16.

Teixera Soares, Rogers (2009): As Associações Médico-Espíritas. Ciência e Espiritualidade em Um Só Paradigma. *Revista Eletrônica de Ciências Sociais* 3(6): 169–189.

Terra, Ronaldo (2011): *Fluxos do Espiritismo Kardecista no Brasil. Dentro e Fora do Continuum Mediúnico*. Marília, Faculdade deFilosofia e Ciências: Dissertation.

Theissen, Anna J. (2006): Spiritismus und Psychiatrie in Brasilien. Eine Anthropologische Perspektive. In: Ernestine Wohlfart & Manfred Zaumseil (eds.): *Transkulturelle Psychiatrie, Interkulturelle Psychotherapie. Interdisziplinäre Theorie und Praxis*. Heidelberg: Springer. pp. 325–330.

Theissen, Anna J. (2009): *The Location of Madness. Spiritist Psychiatry and the Meaning of Mental Illness in Contemporary Brazil*. Ann Arbor: Proquest.

Thiesbonenkamp-Maag, Julia (2014): *'Wie eine Quelle in der Wüste'. Fürsorge und Selbstsorge bei der Philippinisch-Charismatischen Gruppe El Shaddai in Frankfurt*. Berlin: Reimer.

Thompson, James (2020): Towards an Aesthetics of Care. In: Amanda Stuart Fisher & James Thompson (eds.): *Performing Care. New Perspectives on Socially Engaged Performance*. Manchester: University Press. pp. 36–48.

Traut, Lucia & Annette Wilke (eds. 2015): *Religion-Imagination-Ästhetik. Vorstellungs- und Sinneswelten in Religion und Kultur*. Göttingen: Vanderhoeck & Ruprecht.

Turner, Edith B. (1992): *Experiencing Ritual. A New Interpretation of African Healing*. Philadelphia: University of Pennsylvania Press.

Turner, Edith B. (2004): The Anthropology of Experience. The Way to Teach Religion and Healing. In: Linda Barnes & Ines Talamantez (eds.): *Teaching a Course on Religion and Healing*. New York: Oxford University Press. pp. 387–404.

Turner, Edith B. (2012): *Communitas. The Anthropology of Collective Joy*. New York: Palgrave MacMillan.

Turner, Victor W. (1968a): *The Forest of Symbols. Aspects of Ndembu Ritual*. Ithaca: Cornell University Press.

Turner, Victor W. (1968b): *The Drums of Affliction. A Study of Religious Processes Among the Ndembu in Zambia*. Oxford: University Press.

Turner, Victor W. (1982): *From Ritual to Theater. The Human Seriousness of Play*. New York: PAJ.

van de Port, Mattijs (2005): Candomblé in Pink, Green and Black. Re-scripting the Afro-Brazilian Religious Heritage in the Public Sphere of Salvador, Bahia. *Social Anthropology* 13(1): 3–26.

van der Geest, Sjaak & Katja Finkler (2004): Hospital Ethnography. Introduction. *Social Science & Medicine* 59: 1995–2001.

van Dongen, Els (1998): Strangers on Terra Incognita. Authors of the Other in a Mental Hospital. *Anthropology & Medicine* 5(3): 279–293.

van Niekerk, Brimadevi (2018): Religion and Spirituality. What are the Fundamental Differences? *HTS Theological Studies* 74(3): 1–11.

Vannini, Philip, Daniel Vaskul & Simon Gottschalk (2012): *The Senses in Self, Society, and Culture. A Sociology of the Senses*. New York: Routledge.

Varela, Francisco J., Evan Thompson & Eleanor Rosch (1999): *The Embodied Mind. Cognitive Science and Human Experience*. Cambridge: MIT.

Velpry, Livia (2018): Looking for the Social Experience of Mental Illness. In: Mônica Nunes & Tiago Pires Marques (eds.): *Legitimidades da Loucura. Sofrimento, Luta, Criatividade e Pertença*. Salvador: EDUFBA. pp. 31–57.

Verhagen, Peter J, Herman M. van Praag, Juan José Lopez-Ibor, John Cox & Driss Moussaoui (eds. 2010): *Religion and Psychiatry. Beyond Boundaries*. Chichester: Wiley-Blackwell.

Vertovec, Steven & Robin Cohen (eds. 2002): *Conceiving Cosmopolitanism. Theory, Context and Practice*. New York: Oxford University Press.

Vigh, Henrik (2008): Crisis and Chronicity. Anthropological Perspectives on Continuous Conflict and Decline. *Ethnos* 73(1): 5–24.

Voss, Ehler (2011): *Mediales Heilen in Deutschland*. Berlin: Reimer.

Wagner-Egelhaaf, Martina (2017): Einführung. In: Martina Wagner-Egelhaaf (ed.): *Voices from Beyond. An Interdisciplinary Project*. Würzburg: Ergon. pp. 9–17.

Waldram, James B. (2000): The Efficacy of Traditional Medicine. Current Theoretical and Methodological Issues. *Medical Anthropology Quarterly* 14(4): 603–625.

Waldram, James B. (2013): Transformative and Restorative Processes. Revisiting the Question of Efficacy of Indigenous Healing. *Medical Anthropology* 32: 191–207.

Wallace, Alan (2012): A Science of Understanding the Mind. The next Great Scientific Revolution. In: Emma Bragdon (ed.): *Spiritism and Mental Health. Practices from Spiritist Centers and Spiritist Psychiatric Hospitals in Brazil*. London: Singing Dragon. pp. 156–164.

WHO (2001): *The World Health Report 2001. Mental Health. New Understandings. New Hope*. Geneva: WHO.

WHO (2005): *Mental Health Atlas*. Geneva: WHO.

WHO (2007): *WHO-AIMS Report. Mental Health System in Brazil*. Brasília: WHO.

WHO (2014): *Mental Health Atlas*. Geneva: WHO.

WHO (2016): *International Statistical Classification of Diseases and Related Health Problems. 10th Revision. ICD-10*. Geneva: WHO.

WHO (2017): *Improving Access to and Appropriate Use of Medicines for Mental Disorders*. Geneva: WHO.

Wiencke, Markus (2006): *Wahnsinn als Besessenheit. Der Umgang mit psychisch Kranken in Spiritistischen Zentren in Brasilien*. Frankfurt/Main: IKO.

Wiencke, Markus (2009): Performative Therapie in einem Candomblé- und Umbanda-Tempel. In: Anne Ebert et al. (eds.): *Differenz und Herrschaft in den Amerikas. Repräsentationen des Anderen in Geschichte und Gegenwart*. Bielefeld: Transcript. pp. 199–204.

Wikan, Unni (1991): Towards an Experience-Near Anthropology. *Cultural Anthropology* 6(3): 285–305.

Xavier, Francisco C. (1938): *Brasil, Coração do Mundo, Pátria do Evangelho*. Brasília: FEB.

Xavier, Francisco C. (1939): *A Caminho de Luz*. Brasília: FEB.

Xavier, Francisco C. (1944): *Nosso Lar*. Brasília: FEB.
Xavier, Francisco C. (1973): *Rosas com Amor*. Araras: IDE.
Zanini, Giulia et al. (2013): Transnational Medical Spaces. Opportunities and Restrictions. MMG Working Papers 13(16): 1–35.
Zarrilli, Phillip B. (2015): "Inner Movement" between Practices of Meditations, Martial Arts, and Acting. A Focused Examination of Affect, Feeling, Sensing, and Sensory Attunement. In: Michael Bull & Jon P. Mitchell (eds.): *Ritual, Performance, and the Senses*. London: Bloomsbury. pp. 121–136.
Zweig, Stefan (2007[1941]): *Brazil. Land of the Future*. Vancouver: Read Books.

Films

Assis, Wagner de (2010): *Nosso Lar*. Brazil.
Shyamalan, M. Night (1999): *The Sixth Sense*. USA.

Online Resources

ABRAPE: http://abrape.org.br; last accessed 02 Nov 2023.
AME: http://www.amebrasil.org.br; last accessed 02 Nov 2023.
CURARE: https://agem.de/en/curare/archive/; last accessed 02 Nov 2023.
CURARE CORONA DIARIES: https://boasblogs.org/curarecoronadiaries/; last accessed 02 Nov 2023.
CEI: https://cei-spiritistcouncil.com/; last accessed 02 Nov 2023.
DECLARATION OF CARACAS: https://www.globalhealthrights.org/wp-content/uploads/2013/10/Caracas-Declaration.pdf; last accessed 02 Nov 2023.
DSV: https://www.spiritismus-dsv.de/; last accessed 02 Nov 2023.
FEB: http://www.febnet.org.br; last accessed 02 Nov 2023.
HEARING VOICES NETWORK: https://www.hearing-voices.org/; last accessed 02 Nov 2023.

Interviews & Sessions

Interview 03 Nov. 2015: Bruno, medium and administrator of HEM (Chapter 3).
Interview 15 Nov. 2015: Ana-Paula, ex-patient of HEM and volunteer at CELV (Chapter 3).
Interview 22 Nov. 2015: Taylor, lecturer at CELV (Chapters 4 and 5).
Interview 01 Dec. 2015: Terencio, volunteer and administrator of HEM (Chapter 3).
Interview 01 Dec. 2015: Vincente, volunteer and administrator of HEM (Chapter 4).
Interview 02 Dec. 2015: Elisângela, patient at HEM (Chapter 3).
Interview 13 Dec. 2015: Liliane & Bruno, mediums and volunteers at HEM (Chapter 4).
Interview 07 Jan. 2016: Regina, medium and volunteer at HEM (Chapters 3 and 4).
Interview 08 Jan. 2016: Silvia, volunteer at CELV and HEM (Chapter 3).
Interview 23 Jan. 2016: Danilo, client at CELV (Chapter 6).
Interview 24 Jan. 2016: Melissa, volunteer at CELV (Chapter 3).
Interview 25 Jan. 2016: Juliana, volunteer and client at CEB (Chapter 5).
Interview 25 Jan. 2016: Tereza, ex-patient at HEM and client at CELV (Chapter 6).
Interview 26 Jan. 2016: Isabel, ex-client and volunteer at CELV (Chapter 4).
Interview 28 Jan. 2016: Magali, instructor at CELV and volunteer at HEM (Chapter 4).
Interview 29 Jan. 2016: Osvaldo, medical doctor and volunteer at HEM (Chapter 3).
Interview 12 Feb. 2016: Paulo, medium of Dr. Hermann (Chapter 5).

Interview 18 Feb. 2016: Maria-Helena, instructor at CELV and HEM (Chapter 4).
Interview 19 Feb. 2016: Arlindo, psychiatrist at HEM (Chapter 3).
Interview 22 Feb. 2016: Iotti, psychologist at HEM (Chapter 3).
Interview 21 Sep. 2016: Mike, client and volunteer at GEEAK (Chapter 5).
Interview 28 Sep. 2016: Fernanda, client and volunteer at GEEAK (Chapter 5).
Interview 21 Jan. 2017: Maria, volunteer at CECC (Chapter 5).
Interview 13 Feb. 2017: Alexandre, medium of Dr. Wilhelm and instructor (Chapter 5).
Interview 17 Feb. 2017: Renata, volunteer at CECC (Chapter 5).
Interview 16 May 2017: Sandra, volunteer at GEEAK (Chapter 5).
Interview 13 Jun. 2017: Heike, client of GEEAK (Chapter 5).
Session 18 Nov. 2015: Evangelization with volunteer instructor Regina (Chapter 3).
Session 19 Nov. 2015: Evangelization with volunteer instructor Nadine (Chapter 3)
Session 24 Nov. 2015: Disobsession with volunteer instructor William (Chapter 3).
Session 25 Nov. 2015: Evangelization with volunteer instructor Regina (Chapters 3 and 4).
Session 26 Nov. 2015: Psychographic Public Mediumship event (Chapter 4).
Session 01 Dec. 2015: Disobsession with volunteer instructor William (Chapter 4).
Session 03 Dec. 2015: Fraternal Care with volunteer Melissa (Chapter 3).
Session 10 Dec. 2015: Fraternal Care with volunteer Sylvia (Chapter 3).
Session 16 Dec. 2015: ESDE with volunteer instructor Silvia (Chapter 6).
Session 23 Jan. 2016: Mediumship Training with volunteer instructor Magali (Chapter 4).
Session 29 Jan. 2016: Mediumship Meeting of HEM's Administration Board (Chapter 4).
Session 22 Feb. 2016: Mediumship Treatment by Dr. Alexandre/Dr. Wilhelm (Chapter 5).

Index

Abadiana, Minas Gerais, Brazil 139
academia mimicry 97, 159
acupuncture 48
addiction 50, 60
aesthetics; of healing 2, 8, 12–7, 20, 24, 35, 48, 54, 58, 91–121, 124, 142, 151, 155–7, 160–1
affective arrangements 13, 109
Afro-Brazil 21, 29, 34–6, 38, 42, 47, 49–50, 74, 97–8, 105, 107, 124, 135, 138, 149–50
altered states of consciousness 8, 21, 36–7, 50, 94, 117, 155; of sensory perception 11, 110–1, 113, 117, 151
AME see Association of Spiritist Medicals
animal magnetism see Mesmer
anthroposophical medicine 26, 47
anti-psychiatry 26, 45, 51–2
anxiety 49–50, 66, 110, 115, 128, 133, 136
art therapy 43
ASC see altered states of consciousness
Association of Spiritist Medicals 41, 52, 125–6, 140, 150, 153, 158
ASSP see altered states of perception
autoethnography 2, 5, 23, 92, 120
automatic writing see psychography

Bad Honnef, Germany 25, 140
Bahia; Salvador da, Brazil 1, 4, 36–7, 47, 122–3, 135, 150
Basu, Helene 8–9, 108–9
Bezerra de Menezes, Adolfo 39–41
Bhabha, Homi K. 5, 17–8, 35, 96, 155
Biehl, João 45

Bingen, Hildegard v. 6
biomedicine 4, 6–9, 20, 25, 29, 35–8, 41, 51, 66, 85, 96, 148–9, 154–9
body/mind 3, 7–8, 12, 26–7, 33, 36, 39–40, 42, 92–3, 120, 136, 156
Bourdieu, Pierre 116
Bragdon, Emma 53–4, 139
Brody, Eugene B. 44, 50
Brown, Diana 35
Buddhism 28, 119, 121, 149

Caldwell, Kia L. 47–8
CAM see Complementary and Alternative Medicines
Candomblé 21, 34, 49, 98, 150
capitalism 6, 127, 154
capoeira 138, 150
CAPS see Psycho-Social Assistance Centers
captação 50, 52
Cartesian dualism see body/mind
Casa das Palmeiras 43
Catholicism 6, 32, 69, 80–2, 114, 134, 145, 160
CEB see Spiritist Center Barsanulfo
CECC see Spiritist Center Claudionor de Carvalho or Spiritist Center House of the Path
CEI see International Spiritist Council
CELV see Spiritist Center Light and Truth
chakra 102, 114, 121, 125–6, 128, 137–9, 149
charity 4, 29–30, 32–3, 37, 41, 43, 52, 59, 61, 64, 75, 79–80, 85, 87, 89, 95, 100, 112, 122, 126–7, 131, 136, 140, 142–4, 149, 153, 158, 160

Christianity 6, 26–7, 30, 41–2, 105, 114, 148
chronicity 36–8, 50, 53, 115, 126, 129, 138–9, 149–50
Classen, Constance 110
Claudionor 37, 123, 134–9, 148–50
cognition 12–6, 22–3, 35, 41, 48–9, 51, 64, 71, 74, 84, 93, 96–8, 106–8, 111, 116–7, 119–20, 127, 151, 156, 160–1
Colônia de Barbacena 44
colonial; post-; neo- 6, 17, 26, 29, 31, 154
community care 11, 20, 23, 43, 45–6, 53, 59, 86, 145–6, 150, 156
Complementary and Alternative Medicines (CAM) 5, 7, 9, 11, 19–20, 27, 35–8, 47, 50, 52–4, 59, 65, 82–4, 86–7, 90, 96, 121, 124–5, 136–7, 139, 148–9, 152, 154–6, 161
cosmopolitan medicine see biomedicine
COVID-19 157
cross-cultural psychiatry see transcultural psychiatry
Csordas, Thomas J. 11, 15, 19, 92, 116

da Silva, Luiz I. 47
da Silveira, Nise M. 43
Davies, Andrew J. 29
de-Brazilianization 38, 153
de Oliveira, Inâcio F. 39
decision-making 36, 56, 95, 127, 152, 158
Declaration of Caracas 43
deinstitutionalization 26, 43–4, 50, 60, 82, 157
depression 2, 40–1, 59–60, 66, 70, 80, 111, 128, 135–7, 140, 145–6, 157, 161
Devereux, George 26
disobsession 3, 21, 34, 52, 57, 64, 70–6, 79, 82, 85, 89, 95–6, 98–9, 102, 109, 111–3, 136, 138–9, 143
dissociation 9, 119–20
Dolar, Mladen 108
Douglas, Mary 117
Downey, Greg 119
Dox, Donnalee 14–5
DSV see German Spiritist Association

efficacy; effectiveness 1, 14, 16, 37, 46, 53–4, 85, 92, 123, 154

embodiment 5, 9, 11–5, 22, 24, 39, 49, 74, 92, 94–8, 104–9, 116–7, 119, 129, 142, 144, 156
Emmanuel 33
emotion 3, 6–7, 12–3, 22, 26, 36, 38, 40, 48, 50–1, 54, 66, 76, 84, 93, 97, 103, 108–9, 111, 118, 124, 128, 140–1, 145
empathy 2, 22, 67, 89, 99, 110, 117–9, 121, 144, 156
emplacement 12, 156
empowerment 11, 35, 38, 45, 49–50, 78, 121, 155, 160
enactment 89, 94–5, 98
energetic treatment see passe
Enlightenment 5, 26, 29
enskillment see skill
evangelization 4, 34, 57, 66–72, 74, 78, 80, 86–7, 89–90, 96, 102, 105
Evangelical churches 78, 97, 105, 127, 135, 150, 160
exorcism 3, 14, 71, 79, 95, 105

favela 47, 58, 134, 136
FEB see Spiritist Federation of Brazil
fluids 10, 27, 29, 39, 41, 49, 64–5, 72–3, 78, 80, 87, 92, 96, 99, 105, 126, 128, 138–9, 142, 149, 161
Foucault, Michel 5, 51, 116
Franco, Divaldo P. 1, 39–41, 140
fraternal care; attendance 4, 57, 75–80, 82, 87, 89, 94, 96, 106, 109, 111, 139, 141, 152
Frederik 37, 123
Fritz 36, 123

GEEAK see Spiritist Study Group of Allan Kardec
gender 2, 8, 14, 27, 30–1, 35, 44, 48, 53, 59, 62, 112, 128, 159
German Spiritist Association 140–2
Giumbelli, Emerson 33–4
global health 6–7, 9, 11, 41, 156–7
globalization 2, 6–7, 9, 10, 19–20, 22, 25, 32, 37, 75, 124–5, 141, 144, 151–2, 155–6
Greenfield, Sidney M. 36–8, 94–6, 151

habitus 16, 51, 79, 89, 93, 97, 107, 116–7, 131, 141, 151, 156
hallucination 12, 70, 79, 88
Hans 37, 122

health markets 4, 10, 12, 20, 35, 37–8, 44, 156
health policy (politics) 4–7, 9, 42–50, 60, 82, 84–5, 96, 136, 148, 152, 157
health-seeking behavior 1, 3–5, 7, 12–3, 18, 20, 36, 50, 78–9, 123, 149
HEM *see* Spiritist Hospital of Marília
Hermann 37, 123, 130–4, 148–9
Hess, David J. 3, 35–6, 50, 150
Hinduism 28
holism 1–2, 7, 25, 36, 48, 50–1, 83, 102, 123, 154, 158
homeopathy 47, 126, 130
homosexuality 159–60
hospital mimicry 14, 74, 96–7, 138, 151
Howes, David 12, 16, 104, 110
hypnosis 94, 110

IBGE 35
ICD-10 *see* International Statistical Classification of Diseases and Related Health Problems
idioms of distress 49, 93–4, 125, 149
Ilheus, Bahia, Brazil 37, 123
IMF *see* International Monetary Fund
Indigenous 6, 11, 21, 29, 32, 34–5, 42, 47, 58, 107, 123, 138, 157
individual/dividual 1–3, 7–8, 14, 19, 26–30, 35–6, 40, 48, 52, 89, 93, 108, 117–8, 155–6
industrialization 27
inequality 2–3, 32, 44, 47, 74, 96, 150, 157–8
Ingold, Tim 15–6, 119
inner reform 52, 111, 125, 141, 146
insomnia 49, 69, 116
Integrative Mental Health 44–5, 53, 139
International Monetary Fund 44
International Spiritist Council 125, 140
International Statistical Classification of Diseases and Related Health Problems 87
interoception 16, 119, 121
Itabuna, Bahia, Brazil 4, 37, 123, 134–6, 147, 149–50, 157
Itacaré, Bahia, Brazil 135

João de Deus; John of God 37, 123, 139
Jung, Carl G. 40, 50, 155
Jung-Stilling, Johann H. 27–8
Jurema 21

Kapferer, Bruce 14
Kardec, Allan; Kardecism 3, 5, 10, 17–8, 21, 25, 28–32, 34–5, 37–41, 49, 51, 54, 56–9, 62, 64–6, 69–70, 72, 76, 80–3, 86–9, 95, 98, 102, 105, 112, 120–1, 123, 138, 142, 145, 152, 159–60
karma 28, 80, 91, 121
Kirmayer, Laurence J. 7, 10, 93, 118
kundalini 126

Leibing, Annette 48–9
Lessing, Gotthold E. 28
Lewgoy, Bernardo 33, 38
Luiz, André 33–4
Lula *see* da Silva
Luz, Madel T. 47

madness 5, 26, 38–9, 89, 109
Mariana, Minas Gerais, Brazil 73
Marília, São Paulo, Brazil 4, 24, 56–9, 125
Marxism 27
Mauss, Marcel 116
medical anthropology 5, 7–9, 11–3, 15–6, 22, 24, 46, 51, 95, 117, 121, 155, 157–8
medical system 4, 6, 9, 13, 152
medical tourism 38
medicalization 8–9, 20, 42, 44, 50, 52, 89–90, 154, 156
meditation 16, 33, 103, 120, 138, 141
mediumship 2–5, 8, 11–2, 16–7, 21–3, 25–32, 34–7, 39, 49–50, 53–4, 57, 64–5, 68–75, 77–84, 86–9, 91–103, 107–23, 125–39, 141–52, 156, 158, 161
mental hygiene 40–2
Mesmer, Franz A.; Mesmerism 27–8, 30, 128
migration 5, 7, 17–8, 20, 28, 124, 139–48, 152
mindful body 12, 15
mindfulness 16, 119–21, 146, 156
Montero, Paula 34–5
Moreira, Andrei 1–2, 140, 153
Motta, Roberto 35
multiple personality disorder 8
Munari, Luciano 41
Munich, Germany 4, 139–48

Neoplatonism 27
nervos 49
neuro-anthropology 16, 97
neurosis 40
New Age 5, 25, 29, 33, 35, 37, 102, 140, 144, 149
NGO see non-governmental organization
Nichter, Mark 13, 16, 93
non-governmental organization 3, 44
North America 1, 3, 11, 25, 27, 47, 53, 95, 139

obsession 3, 21, 38–40, 65, 69, 71–2, 79, 80, 88, 92, 95, 97, 111, 113, 117–8, 125–6, 128, 130, 136, 148, 158
occultism 29
occupational therapy 45, 59–62, 80, 82, 89
other; othering 8, 15–7, 23, 35, 77, 89–121, 123, 155–6, 161

panic attacks 111
passe 3–4, 27, 39, 49, 52, 57, 62–8, 72, 75–82, 85–8, 94, 96–7, 102–6, 112–6, 122, 125–6, 128, 130–1, 133, 136–9, 141–4, 151–2, 157–8, 161
pathologization 20, 49, 52, 156
Pentecostalism see Evangelical churches
performance 2, 8, 13–7, 21–2, 35–7, 41, 48, 51, 74, 92, 94–8, 108–9, 117, 123, 150–1, 155, 159
perispirit 3–4, 27, 37, 40–1, 64–5, 93, 102, 118–21, 126, 130, 133, 136
person; personhood 3, 6, 8, 13, 18, 20, 26–7, 39, 93, 116–8, 140
Pestalozzi, Johann 30
phenomenology 12, 22, 24, 92
phytotherapy 35, 47, 131, 149, 151
Pink, Sarah 22–3, 110
positivism 10, 28, 41
possession 3, 8, 50, 79, 98, 108–9, 155
Prandi, Reginaldo 37
Psycho-Social Attention Centers 43–7, 59
psychography 32, 34, 40, 76–7, 82, 91, 98–9, 112–5, 128
psychosis 12, 40, 59–60, 70, 106, 128
psychotherapy 25, 53, 81, 83, 93, 118–9
public health 7, 34, 37, 48, 52, 59–60, 80, 84–5, 136–7, 149–50, 154–7

Rabelo, Miriam C.M. 49, 104
racism 6, 34, 51, 159–60
Reiki 33, 126
reincarnation 3, 25, 28–30, 32, 40, 74, 80, 91, 118, 121, 159
rite of passage 95
ritual drama see social drama
Rivail, Hippolyte L.D. see Kardec
Rocha, Christina 37–8, 94, 123–4
Rousseau, Jaques 30

Saad, Manoel 70, 75, 100
Scheper-Hughes, Nancy 116
schizophrenia 8, 12, 40, 60, 84, 98, 109
Schmidt, Bettina E. 8, 98
science mimicry see academic mimicry
self; selves 1, 6–9, 11–2, 14–8, 23, 25, 30, 33, 35–7, 41–2, 51, 67–70, 78–9, 82–121, 123, 127, 140–1, 144, 146, 151–2, 154–6, 160–1
Seligman, Rebecca 98
sixth sense 2, 16–7, 25, 28, 94, 107, 110–6, 119
skill 6, 12, 15–6, 18, 28, 31–2, 48, 70, 91, 100, 102, 105–6, 109, 111, 115, 119, 121, 136, 141, 143, 148, 151
social drama 14, 37, 51, 95
socialism 29–30
somatic; modes of attention 4, 14, 41, 50, 98, 110, 115, 118, 126, 133
somnambulism 29
Spiritist Center Barsanulfo, Marília, São Paulo, Brazil 4, 126–30, 134, 137
Spiritist Center Claudionor de Carvalho, Itabuna, Bahia, Brazil 4, 134–9, 147, 157
Spiritist Center House of the Path, Araraquara, São Paulo, Brazil 130–4
Spiritist Center Light and Truth, Marília, São Paulo, Brazil 4, 59, 70, 75–82, 87–9, 91–2, 96, 102–3, 105–6, 111, 115, 117–8, 121, 123, 125–6, 131, 134
Spiritist continuum 34
Spiritist Federation of Brazil 1, 31, 33–4, 38–9, 125, 140, 150, 158
Spiritist Hospital André Luiz, Belo Horizonte, Minas Gerais, Brazil 51–4
Spiritist Hospital of Marília, Marília, São Paulo, Brazil 4, 56–7, 59–75, 79–80, 82–9, 96, 98–103, 105–6,

111–5, 117–8, 121, 123, 125, 131, 134, 157–8, 161
Spiritist psychiatry 26, 50–4
Spiritist Study Group of Allan Kardec, Munich, Germany 5, 142–8, 152, 156
spiritual ambulance 74
spiritual hospital 34, 74, 85, 87, 113, 129, 138
spiritual progress 3–4, 29–32, 40, 53, 65–7, 73, 82, 87–8, 91, 96–7, 127, 129–30, 133, 137, 144, 147, 159
spiritual surgery 4, 37, 126, 128, 138
Spiritualism 26–9, 31, 118, 121
Stevenson, Ian 1, 25
stigma 43, 45, 60, 65, 79, 82, 84, 87–8, 97, 154, 160
structural violence 2, 29, 32, 47, 147, 150, 154, 158–60
study groups 4–5, 57, 64, 70, 75, 79–83, 87, 96–7, 102, 105–6, 111, 136, 138, 142, 144–6, 152, 161
subtle body *see* perispirit
SUS *see* Unitary Health System
symbolism 8, 10, 13–6, 36, 48, 50, 94, 96, 121, 124, 151

TCM *see* Traditional Chinese Medicine
technology of the self 16, 25, 89, 93–4, 97, 104, 110, 116–7, 152, 156
Theissen, Anna J. 51–4, 87, 150
theosophy 29
Traditional Chinese Medicine 47

trance 1, 26, 28, 50, 101, 106, 109, 129, 155
transcultural psychiatry 7, 36, 125
translocal relations 4–5, 11, 17–20, 23–31, 33, 38, 41, 53–4, 80, 121–53, 155–6, 158
trauma 18, 20, 40, 51, 68, 95
Tucker, Jim B. 25
Turner, Edith B. 15, 92
Turner, Victor B. 14, 51

Uberaba, Minas Gerais, Brazil 39
Umbanda 21, 34–5, 101, 123, 140, 150
Unitary Health System 44–8, 59–62, 74, 83, 149, 157
USA *see* North America

Vale do Amanhecer 32
Vargas, Getúlio 34, 44
voices 1–2, 17, 25, 28, 57, 68–71, 76, 78, 82–4, 88, 91, 94, 103–10, 112–3, 117, 121, 124, 127, 129–30, 133, 144, 151–2, 156, 158

whitening 52
Wilhelm 37, 123, 126–30, 148–9, 151
World Health Organization 45–8

Xavier, Francisco C. 32–4, 40–1, 74, 127, 159

Yoga 16, 33, 126

For Product Safety Concerns and Information please contact our EU
representative GPSR@taylorandfrancis.com
Taylor & Francis Verlag GmbH, Kaufingerstraße 24, 80331 München, Germany